Substance Misuse in Primary Care

a multi-disciplinary approach

Edited by

Rosie Winyard RGN, HV, MSc
Addiction Team Leader/Nurse Practitioner
Luther Street Medical Centre
Oxford City PCT

Foreword by

Andrew McBride FRCPsych
Consultant Psychiatrist
Specialist Community Addiction Service
Oxfordshire Mental Health Care NHS Trust

D1382485

Radcliffe Publishing
Oxford • Seattle

Radcliffe Publishing Ltd
18 Marcham Road
Abingdon
Oxon OX14 1AA
United Kingdom

www.radcliffe-oxford.com
Electronic catalogue and worldwide online ordering facility.

_____

© 2005 Rosie Winyard

British Library Cataloguing in Publication Data

A catalogue record for this book is available from the British Library.

ISBN 1 85775 657 6

Typeset by Aarontype Ltd, Easton, Bristol
Printed and bound by TJ International Ltd, Padstow, Cornwall

Contents

Foreword

It is with great pleasure that I 'fast-foreword' you to this multi-disciplinary book about primary care services for people with substance related problems.

Health responses to drugs have been somewhat overshadowed in recent years by criminal justice priorities, but no doubt the political pendulum will swing back towards health when fashions change. Such changing, complex, overlapping and sometimes frankly contradictory government agendas, have led, nonetheless, to a great expansion of diverse services for drug users during the last 20 years. Unfortunately, this has not been matched by services for people with alcohol problems.

In my view, the single most positive step in the evolution of accessible and unstigmatised services for drug users seeking help has been the development of primary care and pharmacy based help.

I would draw a parallel with the delivery of services for another long-term problem, diabetes. When I was training, most people with diabetes were dealt with by 'specialists' in hospital outpatient clinics – not very user friendly, inefficient and expensive. Now diabetes is managed in primary care (unless the complexity and severity of the disorder demands additional input). Practice nurses and some GPs have developed particular interests whilst others are skilled enough to undertake the day-to-day tasks. I would not seek to push any of the possible parallels too far, but, like diabetes, substance related problems tend to last for years rather than weeks and impact beyond the individual into the family. The only agency in existing UK systems which has lifelong opportunities for monitoring and gently encouraging people into healthier lives is primary care. The pressure in most other health, welfare and criminal justice areas is to move towards shorter, more intensive and, heaven help us, 'cleverer' options.

Even in places where primary care involvement in the treatment of drug users is most developed, we are still some way from drug misuse treatment being 'normalised' in quite this way, but progress has been relentless and positive so far. The institutionalisation of drug use and alcohol related problems as 'other' in the latest GPs' contract may yet halt or even reverse these positive changes.

There can be little doubt that primary care is best placed to deal with the physical and mental health needs of most people with problematic substance use. In addition to their high prevalence and chronicity, primary care is where problems usually present and where people are most likely to stay. The evidence also supports this approach.

> Rapid entry into treatment and the duration of treatment … may be
> more important than the intensity of treatment … providers should

consider structuring their programmes to emphasise continuity rather than intensity of care.[1]

The majority of people who drink too much or use too many drugs simply do not want or need 'specialist' help most of the time. Specialists can be defined by their client group, expertise or qualifications, exclusive methods of practice, or a specific organisational structure. Let us examine these possibilities one by one: psychoactive drug use is endemic; 'expertise' is of limited demonstrable advantage; effective interventions available to the majority of professionals and existing organisational systems are probably more a hindrance than a benefit to most service users. Further, there is no unitary explanatory theory for the pleasures of using substances, no single understanding of all the problems associated with substance use, and limited knowledge about the pathways to happier, healthier ways of living with intoxicating substances.

The good news for generalists and specialists alike is that the art of working with people is both the challenge and the pleasure of this type of work, and, generally speaking, the simpler the intervention the better the evidence of efficacy. To be aware of what we know and can do, and equally aware of what we do not know and cannot or should not do, must always be our aspiration. Working with people and their substance related problems requires wisdom, humility, patience and pragmatism; as well as knowledge and skill. In my experience these virtues are valued in primary care perhaps more than in some other professional areas.

This book will be of great value for all those interested in this important area of endeavour, and will contribute positively to attitudes, understanding and knowledge. And I say all of this from the perspective of a specialist. So, forward, onward and upward into the book itself ...

Andrew McBride
Consultant Psychiatrist
Specialist Community Addictions Service
Oxfordshire Mental Health Care NHS Trust
February 2005

Reference

1 Moos RH and Moos BS (2003) Long-term influence of duration and intensity of treatment on previously untreated individuals with alcohol use disorders. *Addiction.* **98**(3): 325–37.

Andrew McBride FRCPsych has been a Consultant Psychiatrist with the Specialist Community Addictions Service in Oxford since 2002. Previously, he was Clinical Director of the Community Addictions Unit, Cardiff and Vale. He has co-edited the introductory text book *Working with Substance Misusers: a guide to theory and practice* for Routledge (2002) and the forthcoming *Injecting Illicit Drugs* for Blackwells (2005).

Preface

This book takes the patient with a substance misuse problem on a journey to meet their treatment needs. Along the way they come into contact with many skilled healthcare professionals and user advocates, all currently or recently working in primary care.

You are invited to 'listen in' to consultations and reflect on your own practice in order to develop new knowledge and share in the skills of these practitioners. The chapters in this edited volume are not designed to be 'stand alone' but rather link together and cross reference to provide a more comprehensive picture of treatment services.

Some of the contributors have never written for publication before, while others have published extensively. All chose to give their time to write because of their commitment to improve the treatment experience of people with substance misuse problems. In addition they wanted to share their perspective of developing primary care services.

Together they provide an example of a multi-disciplinary partnership – the theme of this book – and a very powerful force for change. I would particularly like to thank all the people who enabled this book to become a reality. These include Andrew McBride, Sue Pritchard, Maggie Pettifer and Jamie Etherington. In addition I acknowledge the help and support from staff at Luther Street including Dr Sally Reynolds, Liz Short, Natalie Goodman and all others who provided inspiration, knowledge and advice. I would also like to thank my two sons, Timothy and Matthew, for keeping me in touch with the challenges of growing up as teenagers in the 21st century.

This book is dedicated to all the patients and staff at Luther Street Medical Centre for the Homeless in Oxford, past and present, from whom I have learned so much. They are an inspirational team who together work out a shared vision for the practice to adopt a multi-disciplinary partnership approach to substance misuse treatments.

Rosie Winyard
February 2005

About the editor

Rosie Winyard RGN, HV, MSc is an addiction team leader/nurse practitioner at the Luther Street Medical Centre for the Homeless, Oxford City PCT. She is also a visiting lecturer at the Department of Healthcare at Oxford Brookes University. She holds a Postgraduate Diploma in Addictive Behaviour from St George's Hospital Medical School, London, and was formerly clinical nurse specialist with the Specialist Community Addictions Service, Oxford. Rosie has also worked as a Health Visitor in primary care services for over 10 years in Oxford and Leeds.

Luther Street Medical Centre is a specialist primary care practice for homeless people that was established in 1985 in a portakabin next to the Night Shelter in Oxford. This moved to a new building in 1998 that is currently being further extended to accommodate the increasing range of services and growing staff team. The centre is based on a partnership between a charitable Trust – the Oxford Homeless Medical Fund – and Oxford City Primary Care Trust. Addiction nurses are directly employed by the PCT to work in the practice and together with GPs, specialist nurses and social support staff, work together to meet the health needs of homeless people in Oxford as part of the 'Shared Care' scheme. Currently 100 people are receiving substitute prescribing for either maintenance or detoxification but overall there are over 500 registered patients, not all of whom have substance misuse problems.

The practice is the base for visiting psychiatrists, complimentary therapists, hepatologists and podiatrists. It is still located in the centre of the city next to the Night Shelter and nearby hospitals.

Luther Street Medical Centre is a treatment centre for all primary care including drugs, alcohol misuse, mental and physical health problems. It epitomises an inclusive, open-access treatment approach with the fundamental aim of destigmatising issues of vulnerability and homelessness. The centre is managed by a Leadership Team including a GP, practice manager, addiction team leader and nurse team leader, who work closely with the Head of Primary Care in implementing the requirements of a Primary Care Trust – Medical Services (PCT–MS) contract.

The editor's values remain her own, including that non-problematic drug use is acceptable. Nurse-led treatment is an opportunity to develop a wider range of high-quality addiction services according to protocols for care developed with medical colleagues and pharmacists, and regularly monitored and reviewed with PCT and DAAT commissioners. Patients have the right to participate as equal partners in both designing, implementing and evaluating their treatments. These should include opportunities for both abstinence and maintenance with different substitute medications. 'Designer Treatment' can achieve its optimum potential if all the partners are given equal opportunities to contribute to its development in the areas of local primary care delivery and also on the wider policy making stage. The future workforce for both addiction nurses and drugs workers is dependent on the manner in which this is integrated today into RCN, RCGP, NTA and NHS policy making.

List of contributors

Catherine Barnard Siney is a former drug liaison midwife at the Liverpool Women's Hospital. She is currently participating in the training of health-care professionals in Northern Ireland and mainland Britain. She has also edited two editions of *Pregnancy and Substance Misuse* published by Books for Mid-wives/Elsevier.

Richard Bryant-Jefferies is a sector manager for Substance Misuse Services in Kensington and Chelsea within NW London Mental Health Trust, and was previously a GP liaison alcohol counsellor in Surrey. He is author of 11 books including nine titles to date in Radcliffe Publishing's Living Therapy series.

Tracey Campbell RNA, PGDip, MSc Nurse Practitioner, NFA Health Team, Primary Care for the Homeless, Leeds. Previously, a hepatitis nurse working with injecting drug users in Leeds.

Claire Chambers is principal lecturer in health visiting within the School of Health and Social Care, Oxford Brookes University, leading the Public Health Nursing/Health Visiting Programme. She has a particular interest in health inequalities and in encouraging student awareness of diversity issues through teaching and assessment processes within curricula. She has published and presented at national conferences on diversity issues and completed a University Teaching and Learning Fellowship focusing on these issues.

John Chilton has been a consultant nurse in dual diagnosis with Gloucestershire Partnership Trust since 2002. He was formerly a clinical nurse specialist with the Specialist Community Addictions Service in Oxford.

Sue Gardner BSc (Hons), MPhil, C Psych, AFBPsS has been consultant clinical psychologist with the Specialist Community Addictions Service in Oxford since 2001. She is also head of trust psychology in Oxfordshire Mental Health Care NHS Trust. Her previous posts include head of 'CASCADE', a multi-disciplinary, multi-agency substance misuse service in East Berkshire, and district head of psychology in the same area. Sue has also chaired the Division of Clinical Psychology and the Professional Affairs Board for the British Psychological Society. She currently chairs the BPS Ethics Committee.

Aidan Gray is director of COCA (Conference on Crack and Cocaine) and is currently working with organisations such as the NTA, Home Office and RCGP to help develop effective interventions and good working practice.

Jane Gray RGN, BSc (Hons) is a consultant nurse with Leicester Homeless Healthcare PMS, Eastern Leicester PCT. She is also a specialist practitioner general practice nurse, and holds a Postgraduate Certificate in Primary Care. She is chairperson of the Homeless Nurses' Group.

Bernie Halford is the named nurse for child protection with Aylesbury Vale PCT. She is a member of the local area Child Protection Interagency Training Sub-Committee and is a training facilitator. She is currently studying for an MA in Law and Society: Child Protection at Brunel University.

Angela Jones is a GP with a special interest in substance misuse at Luther Street Medical Centre for the Homeless in Oxford.

Duncan Williams is a GP in the Amman Valley in Wales and clinical director of PSALT, Wales' largest primary care provider of substance misuse services. He is also a mentor for the RCGP course and an adviser on the Advisory Panel on Substance Misuse to the Welsh Assembly.

Marguerite Williams is the child protection co-ordinator with Luton Teaching PCT.

Rowan Williams has promoted and developed drug user involvement since 2001. She is seconded to Oxfordshire DAAT from the Substance Misuse Arrest Referral Team Criminal Justice Services (SMART CJS), a voluntary sector organisation providing arrest referral across the Thames Valley. Rowan has assisted in the development of OUT, an independent user-led charity, delivering peer education and user involvement in the south-east.

List of abbreviations

A&E	Accidentxixixixixi and Emergency
AA	Alcoholics Anonymous
ACPC	Area Child Protection Committee
ADHD	Attention Deficit Hyperactivity Disorder
AUDIT	Alcohol use disorders identification test
BACP	British Association for Counselling and Psychotherapy
BAI	Beck anxiety inventory
BDI	Beck depression inventory
BME	Black and minority ethnic communities
BMI	Body mass index
CaFCaSS	Child and Family Court Advisory and Support Services
CAT	Cognitive analytic therapy
CBT	Cognitive behavioural therapy
CHD	Coronary heart disease
CMHT	Community Mental Health Team
D(A)AT	Drug (and Alcohol) Action Team
DANOS	Drug and Alcohol National Occupational Standards
DAST	Drug abuse screening test
DEA	Drug Enforcement Agency
DIP	Drug interventions programme
DoH	Department of Health
DTTO	Drug Treatment and Testing Order
DVT	Deep vein thrombosis
EMIS	Electronic Medical Information System
ETO	Enhancing treatment outcomes
FAE	Foetal alcohol effects
FAS	Foetal alcohol syndrome
FAST	Fast alcohol screening test
GCP	Graded care profile
GMC	General Medical Council
GMS	General medical services
GP	General practitioner
GPSI	General practitioner with a special interest
GUM	Genito-urinary medicine
HADS	Hospital anxiety and depression scale
HEA	Health Education Authority
HIV	Human immunodeficiency virus
ICAS	Independent Complaints Advocacy Service

iu	international units
IUGR	Intrauterine growth retardation
JCVI	Joint Committee for Vaccines and Immunisations
LAT	Local Authority Trust
LES	Locally enhanced service
LFT	Liver function test
LGDF	Local Government Drug Forum
LHB	Local Health Board
LSCB	Local Safeguarding Children's Board
MET	Motivational enhancement therapy
NA	Narcotics Anonymous
NES	Nationally enhanced service
NFA	No fixed abode
NHS	National Health Service
NMC	Nursing and Midwifery Council, formerly the UKCC
NTA	National Treatment Agency
NTORS	National Treatment Outcome Research Study
OUT	Oxfordshire User Team
PALS	Patient Advisory and Liaison Services
PCO	Primary care organisation
PCR	Polymerase chain reaction
PCT	Primary Care Trust
PHCT	Primary Health Care Team
PMS	Personal medical services
RCGP	Royal College of General Practitioners
RCN	Royal College of Nursing
RMN	Registered mental nurse
RNA	Ribonucleic acid
RRP	Reciprocal role procedures
SCMG	Shared care monitoring group
SCODA	Standing Conference on Drug Abuse
SFT	Solution focused therapy
SMMGP	Substance Misuse Management in General Practice
ST	Systemic therapy
STI	Sexually transmitted infection
TSF	Twelve step facilitation
UKCC	United Kingdom Central Council, now the NMC

CHAPTER 1

The policy context for substance misuse services in primary care

Duncan Williams

What's happening to primary care?

On 1 April 2004 GPs signed up to a new national contract to provide primary care within the National Health Service (NHS) via the organisation of practice teams rather than the historical individualised and hierarchical mechanisms of personal medical lists.[1] The new contract challenges the team to provide a quality health agenda and offers incentives and opportunities to develop innovative approaches to care. This chapter discusses ideas relevant to current primary care which can be adapted within your practice to facilitate your professional development in the field of substance misuse. This will enable us to maximise more quality options for our patients. You are strongly recommended to follow the learning approach found in the Royal College of General Practitioners (RCGP) certificate in Substance Misuse course and develop your own portfolio of experience, critical reading skills and reflective learning technique.

The following is a checklist of primary care principles.

- It exists in the real world.
- It is local.
- It is accessible and realistic.
- It is long term.
- It takes a 'full-length feature film look' at people's lives in the context of their health.
- 'Snapshots', although useful, belong more in rescue medicine than planned holistic management of chronic health problems which is the strength of primary care.
- It needs to be patient centred but often it isn't.

Stop here

- In your practice, are you confident you apply these principles to your patients with substance misuse problems?

Continued

- Could you pick up one of your existing cases and quickly establish:
  - the initial treatment goals
  - the motivational factors for behavioural change
  - the actions to be taken if review reveals unmet need or variance from direction of progress?

Contracts in context

The new *General Medical Services (GMS) Contract* (2003) is the mechanism by which the government contracts for primary care services from general medical

---

Box 1.1   Changes in substance misuse work after the new GMS contract

Pre-2003/4	Post-2003/4
GPs have individual lists of patients	Patients are registered with a practice, the individual list system is abandoned
GPs cannot opt out of any aspect of patient care without providing onward referral	GPs can opt out of any care defined in the contract as non-core work (substance misuse is defined as non-core)
Substance misuse services are not directly commissioned by primary care trusts, health authorities, etc.	Substance misuse services must be commissioned by the primary care trust (PCT) (England) or local health board (LHB) (Wales)
No particular payments available to GPs providing substance misuse services	Practices are paid for providing enhanced services – substance misuse work (done properly) is an enhanced service
No clear mechanisms to support innovative substance misuse posts in primary care but outside practices	PCTs and LHBs can provide salaried posts to provide primary care substance misuse services
GPs responsible for primary care of registered patients 24 hours a day, seven days a week, 365 days a year	LHBs and PCTs responsible for out-of-hours provision of all primary care
Inflexible staff pay reimbursement schemes make innovative appointments difficult and cumbersome	Global sum payment system to practices would seem to offer opportunities for innovative staff appointments

practitioners, on behalf of the nation. This provides the framework for organisation of all primary care, both directly within practices and indirectly, including non-directly employed staff included in their practical working arrangements.

Historically since the inception of the NHS, general practitioners (GPs) and their employed staff have contracted with the government of the day to provide GMS via a national contract. Fundholding in the 1990s gave budgets directly to practices to manage the interface between primary and secondary care for non-acute healthcare, although GPs continued to be paid contractually via the GMS contract. Fundholding was abolished in 1997, during the first term of the Labour government. A new contract was offered to practices who wished to have a variance on the nationally agreed GMS contract and a number of pilot schemes were established in 1998, these personal medical services (PMS) contracts now form 40% of the contractual arrangements between GPs and the NHS.[2] Personal medical services contracts allow practices in areas of particular need to be paid for organising care along different lines to the standard GMS contract. This enables the practices to take into account any particular local needs, e.g. practices offering services to the homeless, the elderly, nurse-led services, etc.

The new contract introduced in April 2004 relates to the GMS contract. Pilot PMS schemes ended in March 2004 and PMS is now a permanent alternative to new GMS. Personal medical services contracts have not changed as a result of these new contracts but there are variations including 'PCT-MS', 'PMS plus' and 'Specialist PMS'. These innovative schemes will allow providers to specialise in areas of care at a primary level (i.e. accessible and long term) without the provider being expected to deliver the totality of essential primary care. The important changes of the new GMS contract in the context of substance misuse work compared to the previous one are shown in Box 1.1.

Box 1.2 illustrates the changes to patient handling that occurred as a result of the new GMS contract.

Box 1.2   Example of change in patient handling

On 31 March 2004, JB attended his GP surgery looking for help with his heroin addiction. The receptionist said 'Our list is full. We don't want your sort here. Come back tomorrow'.

On 1 April 2004, JB went to his primary care practice and read the notice about the new nurse-led substance misuse assessment and prescribing service. He asked the receptionist if he could enrol and was given a cup of tea and asked to return next week.

Stop here

- Did you attend all those practice development meetings last year?
- Did you plan for this enormous shift in attitude?

The access agenda

> Substance misuse patients without access to services die on waiting lists – an untenable disgrace![3]

Governments and NHS policy makers of all political hues trumpet rapid access to services as a key target for the NHS.[4] (Indeed few professionals would disagree with this aspiration.) However the increase in funding and staff needed to deliver rapid access has not been forthcoming, e.g. 24-hour waiting times to be seen by a GP. Much recent effort has been focused on improving systems of access and flexibility.

Many practices have undergone extensive restructuring and retraining programmes with the express purpose of providing rapid access for patients to the appropriate team member best able to meet their needs.[5] The GP is perhaps best placed to provide investigative and diagnostic skills. The practice nurse could lead on disease management skills, treatment compliance and patient motivating skills, and disease or chronic condition monitoring. The health visitor could lead on primary prevention and child and adolescent mental health.

- What is your practice doing about access?
- Are you involved in the processes of change? (If not why not?)
- Do you have untapped potential?
- Is your team aware of it? Do you need to speak with the practice manager today?

Innovation and service development

Primary care is the melting pot for innovation and organisational experimentation. It is made up of individuals in small teams, with regular contact and interaction between members, many of whom have intimate and long-term knowledge of the families and circumstances of our patients. Team meetings are a feature of good primary care arrangements and these lend themselves to discussion and planned change, critical case analysis, near misses and hot topic discussions. All these are familiar concepts to the committed primary care enthusiast.

Box 1.3 illustrates a system failure.

Box 1.3

JB attended his GP two years ago to ask for treatment for his heroin addiction and was told he'd be referred to the local hospital trust – on 1 April he is still on the waiting list.

The development of local services for substance misusers depends upon individuals prepared to challenge the status quo in their own practice environment and to embrace change as an opportunity to provide something new that currently doesn't exist.

Some ethical issues for continuing debate

How do we view substance misuse activity as a society?

- Is it an illness?
- Is it a behaviour type?
- Is it socially determined?
- Is it culturally determined?
- Does its solution lie within health, education, social policy, or criminal justice?

Are our national treatment guidelines informing policy makers or is it all a bit *ad hoc*? The reader will find when reviewing simpler publications such as *The Orange Guidelines* and reflecting on existing national and local policy that conflict is rife between what we know works in treatment and what is available to our patients.[6] Professional ethics, General Medical Council (GMC) and Royal College of Nurses (RCN) good practice seem to exist as small oases in the desert of substance misuse services. At a whim patients are denied choices, options, treatments and the right to get it wrong.

Stop here

Do you know someone to whom these things have happened, or who has caused these things to happen? It's about time our 'caring' professions really started to care.

Ethical treatment dilemmas

What are we dealing with here? Is this process of risk management in the context of behavioural change? Is the harm minimisation agenda just a smokescreen for continuing the medicalisation of a problem which could arguably be better served by viewing addictive behaviour as dedicated behaviour? Should we be seeking to normalise dedicated drug use and understand its roots in non-pharmacological or neurobiological ways?[7]

What are the areas for development of practice-based treatments and do we have clear national agreement on defining Substance Misuse Enhanced Services in primary care? At the time of writing the RCGP has a clear view on the quality agenda, but local primary care organisations (PCOs) and LHBs seem to be accepting widely differing quality outcomes.

How should services be funded?

The policy context must include reference to the political as well as the health agenda. Is this a matter for health or criminal justice? There is a current drive towards moving funding streams to the criminal justice system via the community safety partnerships. We must be vigilant at this time and press policy makers and commissioners of substance misuse services to measure carefully whether defining substance misuse work in primary care as a non-core activity leads to greater or lesser opportunity and choice for our patients.

- Are you clear on the policy directions from the National Treatment Agency, the community safety partnerships, and the local action teams?
- How will this affect your local service and planned developments?

How can I get involved?

> So where do you go to my lovely, now you're alone in your learning portfolio, tell me the thoughts that surround you – I want to get inside your head – yes I do!
>
> (with apologies to Peter Starstedt)

Now the scene of the practice committed to the new health agenda for all has been set, the following checklist can be used to ensure the knowledge to apply the skills and attitudes most effectively is present.

Pure learning

- *Critical reading skills*: many of the relevant websites teach this, www.cebm.net/courses.asp
- *Scientific evidence base*: RCGP course literature and references.
- *Critical listening skills*: overt/covert mentoring.
- *Audit with a friend.*
- Visit a local service.
- Spend a session surfing the net, there are e-guidelines, websites for Methadone Alliance, Local Street Agencies, User Groups, SMMGP, SCODA, DANOS, and the NTA.

Applying what has been learnt

Once nurses have completed the experiential and evidenced learning, evidence shows they are most adept at transferring their knowledge into practice.[8] Policies and protocols of robust and utilitarian quality can be developed, thus facilitating effective change and new practical innovation. Nurses are also the most likely team members to have already put effective audit into practice in other areas such as diabetic, hypertensive and asthma management.

The team and the agenda for change

Take a look at your team and consider how it operates, do any of the following models apply?

Autonomous care

This is where the practitioner provides case management with reference to their personal knowledge of the current evidence for the management of that condition, e.g. acute management of simple tonsillitis – GP is responsible and may or may not prescribe antibiotics.

Hierarchical care

This operates in a similar way to autonomous care but the responsible practitioner delegates on-going care to another member of the team, either directly employed or seconded to work there. The delegated staff member shares the responsibility in so far as their own training and expertise can allow, e.g. on-going chronic disease management for diabetes mellitus within an agreed protocol between a GP and a nurse practitioner or practice nurse. The GP and nurse retain responsibility.

Shared care – contracted

This is where a number of practitioners who have different expertise share the responsibility of caring for and managing patients, depending on the needs of the patient at any given time. This may be through pre-determined protocols. It is important to note that in the case of prescribed treatment for patients within the NHS, accountability and responsibility is always with the prescriber. (This is a fundamental medico-legal practical point, sometimes not fully understood by well meaning, non-prescribing team members.)

Shared care – *de facto*

This model is similar to contracted shared care but is not formally agreed. This type of approach often precedes a contracted shared care approach.

Delegated

This is where a GP allows another suitably trained and qualified professional to undertake management of patients within a protocol, without the GP having direct contact with the patient. The other professional is therefore delegated the task of case management within a protocol. The GP retains the clinical responsibility as the main author of the protocol.

Principles of delegation

Delegation in primary care is common practice. It is surprising how often new members to the primary care team have difficulty with the concept as described above (particularly if steeped in a tradition of hospital protocols). In reality it is probably impossible to provide current best practice in most areas of chronic condition management without delegation.

Effective delegation means the person to whom a job is delegated is trained to do the job to the standards expected by the governance bodies of both professionals. In addition, the person is confident in their ability to take on the delegated task and is competent to perform to objective standards. Delegation should be supported by on-going appraisal and re-accreditation system to the standards of the governance bodies of both professionals.

Who are the members of your team?

The following is a list of typical primary care team members.

- GP
- manager
- nurse
- pharmacist
- nurse practitioner
- health visitor (HV)
- midwife
- healthcare assistant
- nursing assistant
- patient
- expert patient.

Stop here

- Draw up an exhaustive list of your team.
- Case management in a team context: Consider the team in the context of patients presenting with substance misuse problems and develop a system of managed care based on the models of care – *see* page 17. Include the principles of delegation, where accountability is clearly defined at all levels. Agreed protocols will inform referral pathways and actions to be taken in the light of changing circumstance and variance of patient need.

Working with locality frameworks

The following organisations and services are examples of local provision.

- Practice with its enhanced service contract
- Supervised methadone/Subutex schemes at local pharmacies
- Other local PMS/GMS practices with GPSI
- Local trust arrangements – psychiatric services and secondary care drug services
- Community safety partnerships
- Local active partners, e.g. LATs, non-statutory agencies, probation and DTTOs.

Stop here   Locality frameworks

- Write your own local lists.
- Construct a flow diagram for JB (*see* Box 1.2, page 3) to get help.

Many localities in England (not Wales) have local shared care monitoring groups (SCMGs). Contact your local primary care organisation (PCO) or trust to get involved. If there isn't one find out how they propose to introduce enhanced service payments for substance misuse services in the locality. At the time of writing very few PCOs in England or local health boards (LHBs) have implemented enhanced service payment systems.

Introducing and measuring change

Practice IT systems have come on in leaps and bounds. Many have innovative features which allow the planned introduction of new clinical practice with locally selected read codes and local templates for data collection. The practice IT system should be examined and a team meeting should be arranged. A focus group is a useful way to develop an easily audited protocol to get patients in for assessment, diagnosis of dependency, treatment appropriate to need and long-term follow up and monitoring. Visiting websites to examine other practices' audits is a useful exercise. The audit cycle can be planned using the IT system.

Qualities to look for and adapt from personnel resources

* Leadership.
* Enthusiasm.
* Determination.
* Motivation.

Identify the leaders and enthusiasts, the obstacles (personnel and organisational), the motivators and the milestones to be measured as your services develop.

Stop here

Opportunities of change may inform the motivation of your practice.

Health service managers can perform a patient satisfaction survey early on in their treatment. This is guaranteed to be a positive piece of evidence to show that change is both needed and being made in the practice. Can you demonstrate how your new service has broken down previous barriers to care? Consider the involvement of the local community health council or practice patient participation group.

This is an opportunity for all on the treatment side to develop new skills, attitudes and knowledge which may revolutionise your practice.

The development of quality enhanced substance misuse services in your practice offers the management an opportunity to expand practice services and expertise. This can turn a historical problem into an opportunity for practice change and development, transforming a marginalised and challenging group of patients into a positive experience for the practice.

Partnership opportunities for nurses and GPs to develop new skills

GPs can develop skills in:

- behavioural change techniques
- motivational interviewing[9]
- psychosocial aspects of care adaptable to many other elements of the new contract
- learning and explaining interesting neuropharmacology
- getting job satisfaction – the patients are so easy to treat and so happy with a kind approach
- applying the principles of hard science to a socially challenging group with a holistic approach.

Nurses can develop skills in:

- expanding the nursing team within and outside the practice
- developing clinic/protocol-led care of patients working co-operatively with GPs/patient groups/expert patients, local non-statutory and statutory agencies/ drug workers/CPNs
- opportunities in Child Health Surveillance clinics, maternity care, health promotional clinics, well-person clinics, travel clinics, etc. to normalise a marginalised group
- developing co-operative working with professional colleagues, e.g. healthcare assistants (HCAs) drug workers, CPNs.
- developing skills in assessment, treatment models for maintenance, detoxification, relapse prevention, motivational interviewing and behavioural change – getting professionally involved with a group of people with physical, psychological and emotional health challenges who respond extremely well to an empathic, informed approach.

Summary

This is primary care – an accessible, long-term service based in the real world and staffed by real people offering help in a real way to other real people. It has a very attractive mutuality.

Developing behavioural change models involving pharmacological interventions tied to a realistic service users' frame of reference affords an opportunity at this time in the British NHS to pilot principles of care which should inform humane practice development for years ahead. We are humbly grateful to our patients for offering us this challenge.

References

1   *The NHS (General Medical Services Contract) Regulations 2004. No. 291.* HMSO, London.

2   Department of Health, NHS Modernisation Agency and National Primary Care Development Team. *PMS Contracts*: www.natpact.nhs.uk/primarycare contracting

3   'You die before you get help — that's the way I've lost most of my mates'. Heroin addict, BBC Wales News website.

4   Welsh Assembly (2000) *Tackling Substance Misuse in Wales — a partnership approach*. Papers from the Welsh Assembly, April 2000.

5   Warrender S (2002) *Promoting Advanced Access in Primary Care*. Aeneas Press.

6   Deehan A, Templeton L, Taylor C *et al.* (1998) Are practice nurses an unexplored resource in the identification and management of alcohol misuse? Results from a study of practice nurses in England and Wales in 1995. *Journal of Advanced Nursing.* **28**: 592–7.

7   Cohen P (2004) *Bewitched, Bedevilled, Possessed, Addicted: dissecting historic constructions of suffering and exorcism*. Presentation held at the London UKHR Conference, 4–5 March 2004. CEDRO, Amsterdam.

8   Advisory Council on the Misuse of Drugs (2003) *Hidden Harm: responding to the needs of problem drug users*. HMSO, London.

9   Scottish Executive (2003) *Getting Our Priorities Right*. Scottish Executive, Edinburgh.

CHAPTER 2

Practical guide for the addiction nurse in shared care

Rosie Winyard

Introduction

The management of treatments in primary care can sometimes be characterised by hierarchical and traditional approaches. The following discussion is an example of delegated care within a team approach (*see* Chapter 1) where delegation is according to an agreed level of professional competence and bounded by protocols. In this situation, assessment and treatment may be carried out by either a nurse or a GP, provided practitioners have reached the necessary level of competence and have acquired appropriate specialised training.* Ultimately, the strength of a multidisciplinary approach depends on the implementation of care according to clear guidelines and protocols that have been drawn up according to national and local criteria, in addition to effective communication between team members and the primary care trust (PCT) or local health board (LHB).

The addiction nurse is in a unique position to provide holistic care in a primary care setting. However, the extent to which her skills are used still varies widely across the UK depending on local shared care arrangements between primary, secondary and voluntary sector services. More recently, the National Treatment Agency (NTA) has developed a programme in an attempt to streamline and standardise referral pathways with treatment modalities that will impact on the way all addiction nurses operate in their practice environments. Drug and Alcohol Action Teams (DAATs) are charged with implementing this process, called *Models of Care*, that will have an impact on the way services are delivered in primary care.[1] This is currently being revised (Spring 2005).

The nature of the treatment model for patients with addiction problems used in an area depends on the willingness of GPs and pharmacists to become involved in shared care arrangements under a nationally enhanced service (NES) agreement or a locally enhanced service (LES) agreement within the terms of the new GP contract. This often depends on the availability of support from specialist providers of addiction and mental health based in either primary or secondary care. The extent

---

* Currently, responsibility for prescribing treatments still rests with the GP who signs a prescription although the treatment may be designed by a nurse (*see* Chapter 12). However, substitute prescribing is just one part of effective treatment.

of voluntary sector provision also has an impact on the relationship. The complexity of the type of substance misuse issues managed by the addiction nurse can therefore vary enormously from one area to another, and requires a practitioner approach that is highly flexible and specialised to meet the varied requirements of new primary care and service users.

This chapter considers the patient's journey through referral and treatment pathways illustrating the different ways in which the addiction nurse utilises her specialist skills in a primary care environment. For simplicity, the addiction nurse is referred to as 'she' but this is not meant to infer any gender bias.

The following case study highlights some of the advantages for the addiction nurse working in primary care. It may also raise some of the limitations and can usefully be considered in relation to the questions that follow.

Case study:

John has been injecting heroin for a number of years although was able to stop using drugs on a daily basis when he was in prison last year. He is also smoking crack weekly and buys diazepam tablets to help him sleep. He has tried to detox. himself by buying alcohol and is drinking between 12–16 units daily. He wishes to register at your practice.

Questions:

1   If you were John, what would be the benefits of being treated in a primary care setting?
2   As the addiction nurse, what would be your plan for engagement and assessment?
3   What would be your treatment plan, if any?
4   Can you apply any of this model to working in your own practice setting?
5   Would there be any advantages or disadvantages for (i) John, (ii) the professionals involved of working in a more specialist setting?

Case study (continued):

As the addiction nurse, you are able to assess John the following week after he presented for registration at your practice. Before meeting you he has had a full health assessment carried out by the practice nurse and has been medically assessed by the GP. You have also heard his name at practice meetings where all new patients are discussed on a daily basis. The GP has already prescribed John a course of antidepressants to treat his low mood. In addition he is treated with antibiotics for a groin abscess as a result of risky injecting practices, and inhalers for asthma following a routine health check by the practice nurse.

You meet with John for an assessment of his substance misuse. During your assessment, you both agree that a methadone prescription would be the most appropriate treatment at this time to help him reduce his dependence on heroin. You are able to commence a methadone prescription that day with the support of the GP and ask John to return the following day for titration of the dose. In addition, you assess his alcohol dependence, monitor whether he is taking his other medication and assess whether it appears to be effective.

John has already met the practice support worker who is able to help him obtain some temporary accommodation. You are able to ensure progress of his contact with other team members because you share the same IT system.

The consultant psychiatrist visits the following week to review John's medication as he has a history of bipolar disorder and has had a recent hospital admission in the past six months.

Addiction referral, assessment and treatments in primary care

Patient presentations in primary care may be crisis driven, highly unpredictable and multifaceted. Appointment slots tend to be shorter to cope with a high volume of patients. In addition, there may be active outreach or home visits from the primary care practice in an attempt to engage patients who are reluctant to keep appointments. Primary care treatments are on-going and the patient may continue to be treated by another team member even though the problem of their addiction may resolve or be secondary to a pregnancy or child care issue, for example. The patient and often their family may therefore become well known to the whole primary care team and form relationships with a wide number of skilled professionals thus making a rapid return to treatment more likely if they lapse.

This may be quite different from working as an addiction nurse in an in-patient or secondary care setting where caseload management is often more planned, individualised and appointments have to be made and kept before care can begin. In addition the whole focus of time and care in a secondary care setting is on addiction treatment at a deep, specific level, referring any other issues to alternative specialists, e.g. psychotherapists or forensic consultants.

By contrast, in primary care as part of a LES, addiction treatments are linked to the whole package of physical, mental and social health treatments the patient receives and the addiction nurse can become the co-ordinator of them all, if she is the person to see the patient most frequently and can liaise with the rest of the team. There can however be a potential conflict in this specialist primary healthcare team between the desire to contact those people who are difficult to engage in treatments and the need for addiction patients to demonstrate motivation for change themselves by attending appointments and collecting medication regularly. This may sometimes result in a complex management problem, particularly if the patient has underlying mental and/or physical health problems. Effective management depends on clear referral pathways, good verbal communication and IT support. The addiction nurse can be a pivot to encourage patients to access other in-house and more specialist services as they are likely to see the patient regularly while they become stable in treatment. They need to have a good knowledge of the range of options available and also be familiar with the boundaries of confidentiality agreed with the patient when communicating with other agencies outside the NHS. Team discussions and joint team planning and co-ordination are therefore essential features of this way of working with people with substance misuse problems.

The range of specialist services that a primary care addiction nurse is most likely to liaise with include the following:

- housing
- sexual health
- Accident and Emergency (A&E)
- general medical
- mental health
- HIV
- hepatitis C treatments
- social services
- criminal justice services.

Where do referrals come from?

Triage for shared care

Patient referrals in primary care come from a wide range of services:

- direct from the patient
- housing
- GP
- health visitor
- practice nurse
- midwife
- criminal justice agencies
- A&E
- hospital
- secondary care discharge.

Brief assessments can be carried out by any member of the primary healthcare team (PHCT) or trained worker in a linked agency at the point at which the patient discloses a drug problem or one is observed by the practitioner.

Comprehensive addiction assessments should be carried out only by a specialist addiction nurse or a GPSI who has achieved the required standard of experience and training.

The NTA has developed *Models of Care* as a plan for standardising referral and assessment pathways for treatment of substance misuse.[1] Implementation still varies in different parts of the UK, depending on the availability of shared care and/or alternative specialist providers. In addition, agencies have had difficulty in agreeing standardised assessment and data collection mechanisms, but this is improving nationally to meet the requirements of both the NTA and local DAAT monitoring requirements.

Assessment

The practical reality of carrying out an assessment of substance misuse

It is likely that you will be using a predetermined assessment tool that is being implemented in your area designed as part of the *Models of Care* process.[1] In reality it is very difficult to use such tools while still retaining a degree of patient-led consultation. However, this is vital if they are then to become a part of the assessment process and treatment plan. Tools can be useful in helping to identify and record the complexity of factors affecting addiction, including the types of drugs used and the extent of dependency, see for example the ETO tool on the NTA website, designed by John Marsden.[2]

Addiction is now regarded as a chronic relapsing condition. It is often a pattern of behaviours that become a learned way of coping with stressful situations and may be set from an early age in a person's life. Consequently, effective assessment and treatment plans need to reflect an understanding of this unique pattern and use it as a basis for change. If you want to know more about theories of addiction and in-depth analysis of a range of treatments see, for example, *Drugs and Addictive Behaviour* and *Forbidden Drugs*.[3,4]

Assessment is the process that identifies the types of substances used and past experiences of treatment, in addition to understanding the person's social, physical and mental health. Assessment lays the foundation for treatment that will need to be both chemical and psychological. The most significant factor in maintaining opiate, alcohol or benzodiazepine addiction is often the fear of withdrawal symptoms. However, other addictions such as cocaine may present a psychological craving that is difficult to ignore. It is very unusual for there to only be one drug of dependence. Many people experience a transfer of one dependency for another in the course of their treatment. It is important to be aware of this pattern of cross addiction that may occur in the person's life and trigger factors affecting drug use, as they may have a significant influence on a person's treatment plan for the future. People may desire different treatment outcomes that need to be identified at this stage. For some, control of their drug use is the preferred option. Others aim for abstinence.

The patient's perspective

An important skill is to let the patient tell their story at the beginning of the assessment in the order in which they want to tell it and then later transcribe relevant items of information on to the form, or let them complete sections themselves if they so wish. This enables patients to feel they are being listened to and enables the nurse to concentrate on what they are really saying both explicitly and implicitly by observation, rather than answering the next question on the form. It is more likely that they will tell you more and feel they can begin to trust you if you ask open-ended questions, but try to 'let the patient do the talking'. It's what their drug problem means to them at that point in time that is the beginning of treatment and establishing where they are in the cycle of change.[5] Any contact with a patient may be the only one, but don't be tempted to rush in with your point of view and advice giving unless it is requested. In addition drug users may require help with a number of issues affecting their addiction that may need to be tackled at the same time by other agencies, e.g. housing. Chapter 3 provides further information that could be useful in carrying out the assessment process.

The professional agenda

'It's not rocket science' was a phrase I commonly heard used in the context of carrying out an initial assessment. However, I think it requires great skill and patience to be able to manoeuvre around all the requirements of this initial contact in order to meet both the needs of the patient and the NTA. You are dealing with a very experienced patient who knows far more about their individual condition than you will ever read in a book. Patients may have often been told things they don't want to hear in relation to treatment and may easily become defensive. Respect their views and offer a range of future options for discussion of treatments that are:

- specific
- measurable
- achievable
- realistic
- time-limited.

Be honest about what you don't know but remember you do have knowledge and skill based on previous nursing experience that can inform your thoughts and actions.

Risk assessment

Risk assessment is a key part of the assessment process. It includes risk to the person themselves in addition to their family or the wider community (*see* Chapter 11). Reflection with another senior addictions practitioner as soon as possible after your patient encounter can be helpful in developing your knowledge and skills base. In addition you do not have to make independent decisions if you are not sure about a course of action when working in the team context of primary care. Local user group information can be very helpful to provide current advice on harm reduction and advocacy.

Box 2.1   Assessment process checklist

- Quality of patient–practitioner relationship is key.
- Listen to the patient's story – more than one dependency present?
- What does the patient want in terms of treatment?
- Adopt a non-judgemental approach.
- Care planning in partnership with the patient.
- Record keeping.

Performing a 'brief assessment'?

- A 'brief assessment' can be carried out by any professional employed in primary, secondary or voluntary sector service using an agreed proforma.
- Key aims are engagement and planning future care.
- Time needed: 10–30 minutes.

The 'brief assessment' should include:

- a non-judgemental approach, a confidentiality statement
- observation of body language, physical and mental health, intoxication
- listening to the patient's view of their problem and expectations of treatment
- expressing warmth and empathy
- assessing patient's motivation for change
- information on local drug and alcohol treatment services
- offering a range of treatment and referral options
- negotiating options – specific, measurable, achievable, realistic, time-limited
- develop a short- and long-term plan
- risk assessment: arson, violence to self or others, contact with children
- treatment plan and referral options written down and copy given to patient
- worker reflection.

What are the drugs of abuse?

There is a good review of drugs abuse in *Guide to Drugs*.[6] It may be more useful to refer to up-to-date information from websites.[7–10] Local user groups may give you the latest information on the local drug scene and are likely to access other websites used by users to provide information based on personal experience (both positive and negative) of using illicit substances.[11]

It has long been recognised that only a small proportion of people come to treatment agencies for help in relation to the numbers who have tried illicit drugs or consider that their use does not cause them harm or interfere with their daily routine. Historically it was assumed people would come to primary care services for treatment of alcohol or opiate dependency but were very reluctant to disclose misuse of other drugs such as cocaine or other stimulants because they assumed the practice would be unable to provide help. More recently certain primary care services are offering more detailed assessments that reveal a range of drugs misused including those prescribed and others bought over the counter at the pharmacy. Luther Street Medical Centre, Oxford is now the focus of an NTA pilot evaluation of crack treatment services in primary care because of the number of patients using both crack and heroin. Many drugs can be combined by users or synthesised into different compounds. Table 2.1 shows an assessment tool that indicates a way of recording some possibilities but care needs to be taken not to make assumptions – listen to the patient and take into account prescribed and other medication.

Performing 'comprehensive assessment'

- A 'comprehensive assessment' must be carried out by a specialist addictions nurse or a GPSI.
- Key aims are engagement, identifying level of dependency and treatment options from which patients can select ways they prefer to meet treatment needs.
- Time needed: 45–60 minutes (but may not be completed at first appointment).

The 'comprehensive assessment' should include:

- a non-judgemental approach, a confidentiality statement
- observation of the patient – physically and psychologically

Continued on page 22

Table 2.1   Example of part of a planned assessment tool used to triage patients

Problematic drug use:

Substance	Used	No. of days used in past 28 days	Day last used 1 – today 2 – yesterday, etc.	Is this causing problems?	Rank main problem drug(s) (first three)	Route
Alcohol						
Amphetamines						
Cannabis						
Cocaine powders						
Crack						
Hallucinogens						
Street methadone						
Street Subutex						
Heroin						
Other opioids						
Solvents/inhalants						
Street sedatives/ tranquillisers						

Prescribed drug use: (medical treatment of drugs problems only)
(*Give doses, pharmacy arrangements, name of prescriber*)

Pattern of drug use: (use main problem substances only)
(*e.g. daily, weekend only, binge pattern, alone, with other, chaotic polydrug/alcohol use*)

Fast alcohol screening test (FAST):
For the following questions please circle the answer which best applies.
('1 drink' = ½ pint beer or 1 glass of wine or 1 single spirit)

1   MEN: How often do you have EIGHT or more drinks on one occasion?
    WOMEN: How often do you have SIX or more drinks on one occasion?
    Never   Less than   Monthly   Weekly   Daily or almost
               monthly   daily

2   How often during the last year have you been unable to remember what
    happened the night before because you had been drinking?
    Never   Less than   Monthly   Weekly   Daily or almost
               monthly   daily

3   How often during the last year have you failed to do what was normally
    expected of you because of drinking?
    Never   Less than   Monthly   Weekly   Daily or almost
               monthly   daily

4   In the last year has a relative or friend, or a doctor or other health worker been
    concerned about your drinking or suggested you cut down?
    No   Yes, on one   Yes, on more than
               occasion   one occasion

Dependence checklist:

Tick box

Tolerance: Do you have to use more (*main drug*) to get the same effect?   ☐

Physical withdrawal: Do you get sick as the (*main drug*) wears off?   ☐

Habituation: Do you use more and for longer than you intended to do?   ☐

Craving: Do you have a strong desire to use (*main drug*) and find it   ☐
difficult to cut down?

Behavioural adaptation: Do you spend a lot of time getting, using or   ☐
getting over the effects of the (*main drug*)?

Lifestyle impact: Have you given up work, recreational activities   ☐
or social activities because of the (*main drug*)?

Substance related problems: Have you gone on using (*main drug*)   ☐
even though it is causing you physical or emotional problems?

If three or more dependence is indicated.
With physiological dependence indicated: evidence of tolerance or withdrawal (i.e. either tolerance
or physical withdrawal is present).
Without physiological dependence indicated: no evidence of tolerance or withdrawal (i.e. neither
tolerance or physical withdrawal is present).

Adapted from the NTA. Developed by Oxfordshire DAAT.[12]

- expressing genuineness, warmth and empathy
- identification of drugs used, how much, how often and in what combination?
- routes of use including inspection of injection sites
- assessment of dependency and length of time using
- assessment of physical, mental health – current and significant past
- questions about children – if yes, where they are
- assessment of impact of addiction on significant others
- criminal justice involvement – past and current
- risk assessment in more depth (*see* page 159)
- housing
- benefits claimed
- past response to treatments, if any
- patient expectations versus professional expectations – gap analysis
- assess patient's motivation to change
- negotiate a treatment plan
- discuss referral options if necessary
- discuss compliance and what happens if not
- organise pharmacy to dispense medication if necessary
- agree treatment plan and next appointment.

Testing
It is important to confirm the presence of drugs of addiction prior to prescribing for the patient and at appropriate intervals in the future. This can be achieved by both inspection of injection sites if the patient is injecting and also urine and saliva tests. Patients themselves often request this information if they are involved in the criminal justice system to support their treatment plan. Sometimes the results can be a surprise to the patient if for example heroin has been mixed with benzodiazepines, cannabis cut with cocaine or cocaine with amphetamine and can lead to a dealer being caught out. It is important that tests are not a substitute for observations of signs and reported symptoms of withdrawal, as urine tests can be duplicated and saliva testing may only report drugs used in the past 24 hours. The time taken for drugs to be excreted from the body varies as does the sensitivity of the test. Objective testing can include both urine and saliva testing (*see* page 157 for more information).

Various scales can be used to assess the extent of dependency to substances and are often included in assessment tools (*see* Chapter 11).

In addition, in our practice, an alcometer is regularly used in assessment and consultation to check breath alcohol levels. This may affect future prescribing decisions in relation to how a treatment plan is developed, taking into account the need to address both reduction in alcohol and drug use.

Where to after assessment?
The patient's expectation is often that an assessment leads to a treatment that will involve prescribing either for detoxification, titration, maintenance or to maintain abstinence. This does not always have to be the case and it may be necessary for further consultations based around motivation to change or to organise a rehabilitation placement. You both need to be clear by the end of the consultation

about a short and longer term plan for the future and it is now common practice that this agreement should be written down to form a baseline for planning and review. For additional information that should be given to the patient and a further discussion of this topic in relation to advocacy and treatment, *see* Chapter 3, page 37.

Local protocols agreed by the PCT prescribing lead should determine boundaries of the patient/practice relationship affecting expectations of each other, availability and limits of prescribing in primary care, lost prescriptions etc., *see* for example Appendix 3. They should also make clear referral pathways in and out of specialist treatment services including detoxification and rehabilitation. Certain patient populations are often more successfully treated by secondary care than in primary care addiction services and it is important to ensure easy transition for the patient between them. These include people with complex mental health problems, particularly psychosis, pregnancy, young drug users under the age of 16 years, injectable prescriptions for substitute medication and in patient detoxification. However, the reality of primary care working is that patients may fail to engage with an alternative care provider and it can become a 'catch all' service, overloaded with complex cases unless there is both management and clinician support for a throughput of patients in both directions.

Treatment

Treatment includes both psychological therapies and chemical substitute medications. Both are equally important in achieving effective treatment outcomes. The latest NTA *Research into Practice Briefings, No. 5* goes as far as publishing research confirming that the relationship between the patient and the worker is as important as the correct level of methadone in affecting good treatment outcomes.[13] (For a discussion of psychological approaches *see* Chapter 9, page 121. For treatments of crack and cocaine dependence *see* Chapter 8, page 107. For treatment of alcohol dependence *see* Chapter 5, page 61. Treatment of other stimulants or benzodiazepine dependence is discussed by Peterson and McBride in *Working with Substance Misusers*.[14]) The following section includes some key points about titration, detoxification and maintenance in relation to opiate addiction. Similar principles of substitute prescribing can also be applied to benzodiazepines, if treatment is required, converting diazepam to a liquid form for daily supervised consumption in a reducing dose over a period of time discussed with the user.

Prescribing for opiate dependency
Subutex or methadone?

The choice of substitute medication for opiate dependency depends on a number of factors including patient choice but may be influenced by local protocols. If the patient is under 18, not using alcohol to excess or benzodiazepines, Subutex may be the most appropriate drug of choice as it is licensed in the UK for prescribing to this age group. However, it very much depends on the patient's history of drug use, liver function, state of dependence prior to the initial assessment and whether they have already tried a methadone titration or maintenance that has not proved successful. If a patient is mainly smoking heroin or has not been dependent for many months, Subutex may also be the first choice for substitute prescribing.

If the patient has been injecting heroin for a number of years or is dependent and aware their tolerance is increasing rapidly, methadone may be more appropriate as a first-line treatment. Some people prefer to be prescribed methadone for opiate dependency because they are not ready to stop using heroin on top of their prescription. This is more likely to be problematic with Subutex, which acts as a partial agonist on the dopamine receptors in the brain. The NTA has recently published a good review on this topic.[15] The RCGP provides information about Subutex in its prescribing protocol.[16] Whichever medication is prescribed as a substitute, it is important that regular reviews and planning link with prescribing to ensure that the patient's needs are met, taking into account that they may change over time.

The following sections explore the issues around maintenance and detoxification and some implications for prescribing. They need to be read in conjunction with examples of prescribing protocols designed for a patient population of drug users who may be homeless or in temporary accommodation (*see* Appendix 1 on page 171). Each local area will develop its own protocols, based on the NTA guidelines for prescribing, so they are likely to vary in different parts of the country.

Titration

It is important to have observed the patient's physical state of withdrawal and obtained an accurate treatment history prior to commencing titration. Factors that were helpful in assisting treatment in the past can also be indicators of success in the future. Before titration the presence of opiates must be confirmed by objective testing (*see* Chapter 11, page 157). In addition, visible inspection of needle sites compared with a history of injecting behaviour can provide useful information.

Titration is the process of commencing a prescription for a substitute medication that needs to be initiated gradually to balance the withdrawal of the patient's drug of choice. Sometimes patients have already attempted to start this process to treat their opiate addiction by buying methadone or Subutex on the street. A key factor in achieving success is the partnership approach between the patient, practitioner and the pharmacist, as medication should be supervised and dispensed on a daily basis initially to try and ensure it is not diverted on to the street. Addiction nurses have a key part to play in liaising with local pharmacists at the start of a prescription for substitute medication and its subsequent progress, monitoring its effectiveness and any lapses.

There needs to be a level of trust and co-operation whereby the patient feels they can begin to be honest about their level of opiate use in order to make the correct decision about the methadone prescription. Current national guidelines recommend a starting dose of between 30–40 ml/day supervised consumption. This is often inadequate to prevent withdrawal in someone who is using more than £40 heroin per day, so the patient may still feel they need to use some heroin on top of their prescription in the initial titration stages. A plan should be made about how often the patient can be seen in order to plan an appropriate methadone titration. Usually an increase of not more than 10 ml is recommended at each consultation. In our practice patients can be seen daily or every other day so they can quickly be prescribed the recommended therapeutic dose of between 60–80 mg of methadone. In some cases, much higher doses may be necessary – up to 140 mg or more can be used in some primary care practices. Titration with Subutex is usually more rapid and is described in the protocol in Appendix 2.

An important part of the treatment plan is identifying what the patient is looking for, over what period of time and whether they are aiming for abstinence or harm reduction. Both are achievable, but in different ways and titration is the beginning of this treatment process. Joint planning and timing of appointments are very important. Titration is only the beginning of a treatment plan. There needs to be short and long term planning, regular reviews and clear indicators of success agreed by patient and practitioner. This chemical process needs to be complemented by appropriate psychological support.[13]

The type of counselling offered by addiction nurses during consultation varies greatly depending on the practitioner and the patient. Various approaches are likely to be effective at different times. Common elements displayed by practitioners should be the natural skills of engagement including warmth, empathy, a non-judgemental approach, listening and communication skills. Chapter 9 reviews a range of talking therapies and ways in which they can be used by addiction nurses. Most addiction nurses working in primary care would not claim to be providing formal counselling although they may be supported by supervision from psychologists or psychotherapists working in depth with patients in the practice environment. Addiction is often related to grief and loss, so there are benefits to be gained from working together in partnership with other counselling professionals who have more time to focus specifically on these issues in contracted sessions.

Maintenance
Maintenance is the process of achieving harm reduction or stability for the patient so that they can carry on their daily living activities as normally as possible. In some cases this may take many months or years of being prescribed substitute medication for opiate users. One aim is to reduce the need for injecting heroin on top of a methadone prescription. Another is to prevent it all together, if the patient is able to achieve stability. Evidence suggests that an appropriate dose is between 60–120 mg methadone to achieve the greatest benefit.[15] It is important to assess each individual case because of different absorption levels of the drug, responsiveness to the dose and variations in mental or physical health or social circumstances. Partnership working between professionals and the patient should facilitate the identification of specific goals for maintenance that are achievable. In reality there may be frequent transitions between detoxification and maintenance, depending on these goals, but it is important not to confuse the two processes. Patients may begin to use a variety of other drugs for their euphoric effect, in addition to methadone, particularly crack cocaine or benzodiazepines, increasing their risk taking behaviour.

The Criminal Justice Interventions Programme (CJIP) was launched in 2003 (now called the Drugs Interventions Programme (DIP)). Rapid access to the treatment system is identified as part of the prison aftercare system that frequently includes maintenance prescribing with either methadone or Subutex. Advantages of joint working between health and criminal justice agencies have been described for both patients and professionals and can include improved access to both agencies, better retention in treatment, local networking and more financial investment leading to an increased capacity for all in the treatment system. Information sharing can still sometimes be a problem and this is an issue currently being tackled by all the agencies involved. Some treatment agencies remain wary of too many close links on the grounds that it may influence their ability to act equitably for all their patients. For more information *see* www.cjipinfo@coi.gsi.gov.uk.

Detoxification

Community detoxification is the process of achieving asymptomatic abstinence. This can be achieved by the patient taking appropriate medication to reduce the severity of withdrawal symptoms from opiates (*see* Appendix 1). Detoxification from opiates can be achieved by prescribing methadone, Subutex or lofexidine. A combination of dihydrocodeine and diazepam has frequently been used in the past but may no longer be prescribed because of the risk of overdose and diversion on to the streets. It is still frequently requested by patients but there appears to be a lack of good research evidence nationally to support its effectiveness at this current time.

Key factors influencing the effectiveness of community detoxification include the availability of substitute prescribing, counselling, access to healthcare, social support, housing, and a plan both for the process of detoxification itself and for the future. This plan needs to be developed jointly between the worker and patient and should include a range of options that have been considered tailored to each individual case. In many cases, detoxification is part of a process in the cycle of change that may lead to abstinence but may also result in the need for work around relapse prevention.[5] A flexible approach to treatment planning is essential. Motivational enhancement techniques are an important part of this stage in the patient's treatment journey and a non-judgemental, empathetic approach by the worker in order to establish trust between the professional and patient.[17]

In Oxford patients have access to a five-bed residential detoxification unit in a local house provided by Oxford City Council. This project was originally set up with money from the Rough Sleepers Unit to assist people who were unable to benefit from help elsewhere. It is managed jointly between English Churches Housing Group and Luther Street Medical Centre who provide the medical and nursing support around detoxification from drugs. It opened in 2001 and has so far provided help to 61 residents over the time period to January 2004. The average length of stay has been between two and a half to four months prior to moving on to residential rehabilitation elsewhere. Forty four per cent of residents have moved to rehabilitation, 15% have settled in their own accommodation and 15% into hostel accommodation when they have been previously sleeping rough or using the night shelter. There have been a total of 74% positive 'move ons'; 58% of whom were still not using drugs six months later. Part of its success is due to the excellent staff team, close inter-agency working and links between past and present residents who frequently return to share their experiences.[18]

Abstinence

The residential detoxification unit project provides an interesting example of how abstinence can be achieved in a community setting. During the weeks immediately following detoxification there needs to be advice and information around relapse prevention, including overdose prevention as this period is most commonly associated with drug related deaths. Some people prefer to use a complete chemical blocking agent like naltrexone in order to strengthen their ability to stop using heroin. (*See* Appendix 2 for transfer to naltrexone from Subutex or methadone).

Transfer to naltrexone works best if the patient continues to be motivated to maintain abstinence and the drug is taken with the support of a friend or family member. Before initiating naltrexone liver function tests need to be carried out and blood pressure monitored to ensure these are within normal limits.

Achievement of abstinence by chemical means is unlikely to be successful without other behaviour changes in relation to social support, housing or alternative training or employment. It is likely to take months for these changes to be integrated into a person's way of life.

Summary

This chapter has covered a broad area of ground in relation to assessment and treatment pathways. The skills and knowledge base of nurses need to be extensive in order to function effectively in a primary care context, whether working independently, located in a primary care practice once a week or employed directly as a member of a primary healthcare team. The underlying theme that emerges through all this work is that of partnership between professionals and patients and the need to communicate effectively. The future direction for addiction nurses in primary care will be strongly influenced by opportunities arising from new ways of working emerging from the implementation of the GP contract (2004) and *Models of Care*.[1,19] It is up to nurses themselves to promote their skills by using influence locally and nationally in conjunction with the work of their GP colleagues in order to improve the effectiveness of treatment services in primary care for patients. A successful primary care service needs to be supported by the availability of secondary specialist providers to provide training, support for clinicians and time to take on the more complex cases. This is in addition to an appropriate system of referral pathways and a range of voluntary sector services.

References

1   National Treatment Agency (2002) *Models of Care, Parts 1 and 2*. National Treatment Agency, London.
2   Marsden J (2001) *Screening and Triage Assessment for Structured Substance Misuse Services*. National Addictions Centre, London.
3   Ghodse H (2002) *Drugs and Addictive Behaviour*. Cambridge University Press, Cambridge.
4   Robson P (1999) *Forbidden Drugs*. Oxford University Press, Oxford.
5   Prochaska J and DiClemente C (1986) Towards a comprehensive model of change. In: WR Miller and N Heather (eds) *Treating Addictive Behaviours* (2e). Plenum, New York.
6   Drugscope (2004) *Guide to Drugs*. Drugscope Publications, London.
7   Drugscope: www.drugscope.org.uk
8   Harm reduction information: www.hit.org.uk
9   National Treatment Agency: www.nta.nhs.co.uk
10   Europe Against Drugs: www.druginformation.nu
11   Personal User Experiences: www.bluelight.nu
12   O'Brien D (2004) *Planned Assessment Tool* based on ref. 2 above.

13 National Treatment Agency (2004) *Research into Practice Briefings No. 5.* National Treatment Agency, London.

14 Peterson T and McBride A (2002) *Working with Substance Misusers: a guide to theory and practice.* Routledge, London.

15 National Treatment Agency (2004) *Research into Practice Briefings No. 3.* National Treatment Agency, London.

16 Royal College of General Practitioners (2003) *Buprenorphine Prescribing Protocol.* RCGP, London.

17 Miller W and Rollnick S (2002) *Motivational Interviewing.* Guilford Press, New York.

18 Oxford Drug Recovery Project (2004) Steering Group Minutes.

19 *The NHS (General Medical Services Contract) Regulations 2004. No. 291.* HMSO, London.

Further reading

* Seivewright N (2001) *Community Treatment of Drug Misuse: more than methadone.* Cambridge University Press, Cambridge.
* *Black Poppy* (2004) **9**: 9–10.

CHAPTER 3

Users and practitioners: an equal partnership

Rowan Williams

This chapter provides the substance misuse nurse with an introduction to the processes and practice of user involvement in drug treatment. It gives an overview of drug service provision to put the patient experience into context, and describes the following three levels of user involvement.

1 **Patient involvement in individual healthcare**: Two-way communication between nurse and patient using a holistic care planning approach – nurtures good relationships and improved outcomes for individuals.
2 **User participation in service provision**: User feedback on existing services highlights problem areas and good working practice. User participation in service delivery and planning is an invaluable organisational resource that also offers the opportunity for inclusion and personal development to the user.
3 **User consultation in strategic decision making**: On-going user input in the planning of drug treatment provision and policy setting – removes barriers, improves access to treatment and improves quality and choice.

Patient involvement in practice is prioritised and described in depth as it is pertinent to substance misuse nurses in the primary care setting.

User involvement is a bottom-up approach that has many positive paybacks. Non-tokenistic user involvement will increase the efficiency and quality of a service, empower and strengthen the self-reliance of service users, create a democratic and user friendly environment and fulfil policy requirements. The inclusion of user opinions in decisions regarding their own care and in service provision is democratic and equitable.

> Effective patient and public involvement is fundamental to an NHS based on choice, responsiveness and equity.[1]

There is much deliberation about the definition of 'user' in the context of the drugs field. In this instance it is used as a catch-all term to describe drug/alcohol users and ex-drug/alcohol users who have experienced significant problems attributed to their use of substances. This chapter has been written with the help of users. The quotations used are from individuals and are not necessarily representative. Drug users are a heterogeneous population and the comments included are only intended to illustrate particular points.

Perceptions of drug treatment

Drug users have historically been stigmatised, marginalised and subjected to an arbitrary treatment system that remains variable in different geographical areas. In some areas excellent, supportive and innovative drug services exist whilst others lack any provision at all. In recent years, progress has been made in making drug services accessible and responsive to the needs of users. However, negative perceptions, lengthy waiting times, below standard services and poor local commissioning decisions continue to impact upon many users' experiences of drug treatment.

An unprecedented amount of funding has been released into the drugs field since the publication in 1998 of the government's ten year strategy *Tackling Drugs to Build a Better Britain* (amended 2002).[2] Government funding, in the main, has been targeted at criminal justice interventions, however, with integration, mutual targets and key performance indicators, the drug treatment field generally can benefit from the extra capacity created. Increased funding brings increased monitoring and evaluation and users are finally being regarded as integral to these processes.

Guidance is now available to inform the field of good working practices and the emerging evidence base for drug treatment. The NTA has introduced national frameworks to direct drug services and is attempting to standardise the field whilst increasing capacity. Prior to this, drug services often operated in isolation utilising traditionally favoured treatment methods with little recourse to the evidence base. Drug users, on seeking help, were often hindered by the high expectations of the agencies established to support them. The service was prioritised over the individual.

The existence of the now defunct Addicts Index, a national database of drug users that professionals were legally obliged to inform, meant that users seeking treatment were registered as addicts with the Home Office; a powerful deterrent to accessing support. Many factors inhibit engagement with treatment services and these, when compounded by an often chaotic or difficult lifestyle, continue to keep the total numbers in treatment low.

Traditionally, substitute prescriptions and other treatments have been imposed upon drug users. Health professionals tended to assume that they could judge, on the patient's behalf, the necessary treatment, quality of care and outcomes. Moralising and judgemental attitudes were not unusual in healthcare settings and treatment punitive with reduction or loss of prescription threatened for non-compliance. Methadone has been regularly prescribed under the optimum dose. Reduction regimes were widely endorsed due partly to prescribers' fears of unsuitable dosing in an increasingly litigious climate, with users often coerced to strive for the distant goal of abstinence. It is now widely accepted that stability of prescription, and a concomitant stable lifestyle, is more appropriate than reduction for many patients.

Few GPs were willing to prescribe substitute medication to a 'time-consuming' patient group and consultant psychiatrists controlled the treatment system. Specialist drug clinics were often centralised and staffed by mental health professionals. In-patient detox. beds were inappropriately situated in hospital psychiatric wards.

> 'I was the only person doing a detox. on the unit. I felt really rough and totally paranoid. You couldn't imagine a worse environment to withdraw in. I was in the next bed to someone who was a self-harmer and it

completely freaked me out. I left after a day and a half after he tried to set fire to himself.'

Negative images of drug users released as part of awareness raising campaigns by the government and by service providers have demonstrated the fruitlessness of shock tactics. Users are risk takers by definition and often cannot relate to the images portrayed by the government and media. Poor image has compounded users' status as second class citizens stigmatised by UK society and overlooks the fact that drug and alcohol use is probably the largest, and most costly, cross-cutting social issue of our time.

Drug treatment provision is improving but there is still room for further improvement particularly in some areas of the country. A greater range of treatments is being offered, including psychosocial support and aftercare, and quicker access to treatment is generally being achieved. User groups and representatives, with the support of the NTA, are adopting the role of treatment watchdogs and helping to identify and inform good practice.

Box 3.1   Summary

- Users have been stigmatised and marginalised.
- The old drug treatment system was arbitrary and has contributed to negative perceptions.
- Changes and improvements in drug treatment are occurring.

The emergence of user involvement

Over the past few decades drug user activists have fought for progressive legal reform, increased and improved treatment provision and their right to have a voice in decision making.

> Users have been leading change for years. The contribution that users have made is particularly important to the evolution of harm reduction.[3]

The promotion of harm reduction techniques is vital to the wellbeing of users. Safety information (and misinformation) is passed through word of mouth along informal user networks. Through involving users, these networks can be utilised for providing clear and factual harm reduction information and to break down myths.

The emerging concept of user involvement is now incorporated in policy guidelines for the delivery and development of public services. Consumer consultation is becoming firmly established throughout the NHS in line with the *NHS Plan* (2000) which requires two-way communication with patients in the planning and provision of services:

> NHS care has to be shaped around the convenience and concerns of patients. To bring this about, patients must have more say in their own treatment and more influence over the way the NHS works.[4]

Indeed the government now regularly refers to the patient as the 'driver' and new dynamic behind the modern NHS.

Due to rapid expansion of the workforce, employment opportunities for users have increased. Services were adopting a 'two year clean' rule whereby users could not have accessed services for two years prior to employment. These guidelines were updated by Drugscope and the NTA in 2003 and state that drug users should be employed on merit and their ability to do the job rather than on the length of time they have remained 'clean'.[5] Users who are stable on substitute prescriptions can be employed in the field.

User groups and representatives are a voice for change, advocating fair, equal care and treatment. Local user groups are being established nationwide and are at different stages of development. User groups are involved in a diverse range of activities including promoting harm reduction and providing advocacy. Many of these activities can supplement primary care practice. Peer-led activities are usually regarded by drug users as credible, informative and useful.

Box 3.2   Good practice – users campaigning for change and offering support

'Do It Yourself': 'DIY' in Walsall was set up three years ago in response to the need for users to have a voice in treatment. The group is fully supported by Walsall Drug Action Team (DAT) and is proactive in its approach offering support to people affected by HIV, hepatitis C and to parents and carers on an individual and group basis.

Researchers have argued that peer education has considerable strategic value in relation to drug prevention as it offers a route to inclusion for under-represented groups, and utilises existing social networks to provide information, make referrals and/or distribute equipment.[6]

Peer education plays an important role in reinforcing harm reduction messages. Hard hitting messages are articulated with greater impact if related from experience rather than relayed from textbooks.

> 'That experience did not stop me banging up and within three months
> I had another DVT [deep vein thrombosis] in my other leg. I was in
> hospital for about eight weeks that time. Eventually after the third DVT
> I decided enough was enough.'

Box 3.3   Good practice – users delivering peer education and conducting consultation

Oxfordshire User Team (OUT) delivers peer-led workshops on harm reduction to intravenous drug users. The aim of the workshops is to give high quality information on hepatitis C and other bloodborne viruses, overdose prevention and response etc., to encourage user involvement, and to provide a platform from which OUT may consult with users on any relevant issues. The majority of workshop attendees is not in contact with drug services.

Peer advocacy services are increasingly challenging poor practice.

Box 3.4   Good practice – users offering peer advocacy and training

The Alliance is a national organisation offering advocacy to people experiencing difficulties with drug treatment. It has a number of regional advocates who are able to link up with users in their local areas. If this coverage is not available The Alliance advocates from its London base. The Alliance offers training to drug user advocates and on-going support to local user groups practising advocacy. The organisation prioritises user involvement in all its work.

Negative perceptions persist. Many users are still unaware of the changes to drug treatment and the benefits of user involvement. It is the responsibility of practitioners to inform drug users of service changes and developments, and users can assist in this process.

Box 3.5   Summary

- User involvement is firmly established in the treatment agenda and is becoming mainstream.
- User groups are involved in a diverse range of peer-led activities.
- National and local user groups are informing practice.

Patient involvement in individual care

Users' opinions are finally being regarded as integral to their care and user consultation intends to ensure a 'real therapeutic alliance'.[7] The impact of the patient's encounter with drug services can affect their drug use, treatment, social and psychological functioning and quality of life. Good consultation in an honest and non-judgemental process will eradicate negative impact and lead to improved treatment outcomes.

Patients' rights and responsibilities

The rights and responsibilities of patients should be made clear at the outset of all patient relationships. A charter outlining rights and responsibilities should be displayed clearly in all practices and talked through with the patient at the beginning of the care planning process to ensure understanding. The charter shown in Box 3.6 can be adopted and modified according to individual practice requirements.

Box 3.6   SCODA service user's charter of rights and responsibilities[8 –12]

A drug service user has both rights and responsibilities. The service provider has an obligation to make each of these explicit to the service user.

A service user has the right to the following:

- Assessment of individual need (within a specified number of working days).
- Access to specialist services (within a maximum waiting time), and the right of immediate access on release from prison.
- Full information about treatment options and informed involvement in making decisions concerning treatment.
- An individual care plan and participation in the writing and review of that care plan.
- Respect for privacy, dignity and confidentiality, and an explanation of any (exceptional) circumstances in which information will be divulged to others.
- Referral for a second opinion, in consultation with a GP, when referred to a consultant.
- A written statement of service user's rights.
- The development of service user agreements, specifying clearly the type of service to be delivered and the expected quality standards.
- The development of advocacy.
- An effective complaints system.
- Information about self-help groups and user advocacy groups.

A service user's responsibilities to the service provider include the following:

- Observing 'house' rules and behavioural rules, as defined by the service (e.g. not using alcohol or drugs on the premises, treating staff with dignity and respect, and observing equal opportunities and no-smoking policies). Specific responsibilities within the framework of a care plan or treatment contract (e.g. keeping appointment times and observing medication regimes).

Patient/practitioner relationship

Research highlights the importance of the patient/practitioner relationship in achieving positive outcomes. To achieve effective user involvement the dialogue between nurse and patient is paramount and honesty is a key element to this.

> 'Ex-drug and alcohol users always remember the worker who helped them along the road to recovery.'

An open and tolerant attitude should be nurtured. Stereotypical approaches to the problems of patients can act as a further deterrent to treatment entry and retention.[13] Patient perceptions of, and engagement with, programmes can lead to positive outcomes such as those associated with reduced frequency of drug use.[14] Treatment should be tailored to individual need.

Resourcing illicit drug use and using drugs can be a full time activity and initial appointments are often missed for this reason. Attrition rates are high. Significant numbers of users who attend first appointments do not return for a follow-up appointment. This reflects the need for immediacy felt by drug users and their difficult lifestyles, and highlights a need for quicker access to treatment.

> 'It took me ages to get around to admitting I needed help. I was given an appointment in three weeks time. Three weeks may as well have been three years to me – I could not think beyond my next hit.'

A broader understanding of the psychological impact of drug use, local trends and street level knowledge informs practice. The gap between professional and patient is narrowing as the benefits of learning from each other are realised. Patients can impart information and expertise gained through life experience giving real insight to the practitioner.

> 'The urge for crack cocaine completely took over. I would spend hours at a time (probably totalling months of my life) picking up (and smoking) dust and particles off the carpet convinced that I had dropped some crack before I had licked the last pipe.'

Box 3.7   Good practice – user/practitioner relationship

User representatives or groups can offer a 'buddying scheme' where professionals new to the field spend part of their induction period with a user(s) discussing lifestyle and drug issues. Sharing and understanding the perspectives and lifestyles of others is an important part of the cultural shift needed to make drug user involvement work.

Patients' motivation levels are difficult to assess and fluctuate – many different factors lead to successful outcomes for individuals. The factors that affect drug use are often away from the primary care setting, e.g. personal relationships, self-esteem, peer pressure.

> 'I'm gonna stick to my script again when my partner goes to prison next month. I know there's no point trying at the moment 'cos with him around I just can't do it.'

Opiate dependency is a chronic relapsing condition, and few problematic users of any drug manage to give it up at their first attempt. Users can gain from each treatment episode and whilst no research exists on the cumulative effects of intermittent service contact the following quotation supports the view.

> 'I left rehab. after a couple of months but the stuff I learned there stayed with me and helped me when I eventually got my life back together.'

Barriers to engagement and retention

The new relationship can feel threatening to both the practitioner and the patient. Barriers should be identified and explored at the earliest opportunity and may include the following.

- Patients may communicate information selectively in order to achieve specific outcomes, especially if they fear they will not achieve these by being completely open.[1]
- Agendas driven by different values, e.g. criminal justice versus health.
- Patients may lack the skills and information to make informed decisions.
- The patient may choose treatment options that have detrimental effects on health and wellbeing.
- The patient may feel unable to articulate underlying issues due to concerns regarding the consequences of doing so.
- Poor communication from the professional may inhibit user engagement.
- The patient may have a deferential attitude towards professionals.

Enabling users to become involved in their own care can help overcome these barriers, increase satisfaction and is rewarding for both the practitioner and patient. Better relationships will lead to increased trust, self-esteem and empowerment, and should result in positive health effects.

Information and communication

Primary care settings should provide a friendly and accessible environment – users should feel at ease and be provided with plenty of written and visual information.

Box 3.8   Good practice – information

All written resources produced by your service should be created in co-operation with users to ensure readability and a user friendly format.

Use easy to understand language and avoid jargon. The language of the drug field is full of acronyms and terminology specific to the drug treatment system. Users' language and slang is comparatively obscure. Good communication is crucial between health professionals and patients and administrative and support staff.

Give out as much information on treatment availability and outcomes as possible and explain why particular treatment is suitable or unsuitable. Information is vital to inform choice.

Care planning

High importance should be attached to the care plan. The care plan is a contract created and agreed by the patient and the nurse with milestones and goals included. It should be flexible and achievable, regularly reviewed, and amended by agreement. Good assessment, sound protocols and a robust care plan give the patient ownership of their care. Where it is practical and deemed beneficial, carers should also be included in the care planning process.

Sometimes the needs of the patient and individual choice are at odds. Choice is limited by financial constraints, availability and the detrimental impact of some treatment options on the user. It is important to discuss the benefits and pitfalls of treatments with the user and explain the necessity for some arrangements that may be at odds with the patient's requests. For example, explain that supervised consumption of methadone is intended to stop diversion into the black market. Non-supervised prescriptions can be agreed as a milestone within the care planning process.

Working to an agreed patient-centred plan of care allows the patient to take responsibility for non-compliance and credit for achievement.

Complaints and advocacy

Services complaints procedures should be made clear and given to the patient in written format at the outset. A staff member should be nominated to deal with complaints. Information on independent advocacy services should also be made available.

Advocacy is provided nationally by The Alliance and locally by user groups in some areas. Voluntary sector organisations such as the Independent Complaints Advocacy Service (ICAS) will also help. Patient Advisory and Liaison Services (PALS) are now found in every NHS trust, although both ICAS and PALS workers are not often drug specialists.

Box 3.9   Good practice – peer advocacy case study

Karen is a 42-year-old heroin addict, who has been using on and off for 20 years. She stopped injecting one year ago when she started her present methadone prescription. Karen works full-time and this makes it difficult to get to the pharmacist twice a week to pick up her prescription.

For three months Karen has been smoking (chasing) heroin on a daily basis – ever since losing her prescription and not having time to leave work and visit her doctor.

Karen's partner did not know she had been using illegal drugs again but he beat her up last month when she spent some of their savings.

Karen did not tell her prescriber that she was using for fear that her script would be stopped. Karen spoke to a representative of Oxfordshire User Team (OUT) about her situation and was linked to a peer advocate. The advocate supported Karen at her fortnightly appointment where the nurse was genuinely surprised that Karen felt she could not speak honestly with her. Over the next weeks the methadone dose was titrated up to a level where Karen felt comfortable. Karen has not taken heroin since.

Continued

Outcomes
- Karen is no longer using heroin and is complying with a treatment regime.
- The relationship between Karen and her nurse has improved.
- Professionals (nurse and OUT) are alerted to domestic violence and are able to support.
- The risk of accidental overdose has decreased.

Checklist for nurse practitioners

- Have I outlined all organisational practicalities, e.g. opening times?
- Does the patient understand his or her rights, e.g. to complain, to advocacy?
- Are the consequences of breaking rules made clear and are they understood?
- Has the patient outlined their expectations in the relationship?
- Have I outlined my expectations in the relationship?
- Following assessment, has a care plan been devised in partnership with the patient?
- Is the patient following a delineated care pathway?
- Have I discussed all treatment options and given reasons for suitability or non-suitability, and are these understood?
- Have I given out all relevant harm reduction material?
- Have I passed on information about, and contact details for, local user activities?

Box 3.10   Summary

- Users should understand their rights and responsibilities.
- Honest communication between nurse and patient leads to positive outcomes.
- The care plan is a key element of drug treatment.

Patient involvement in service provision

While many professionals support the notion of increasing user involvement in service provision, they are often uncertain as to how to achieve this in practice. To avoid tokenism, users will need to be supported and informed of operational practice at every level, and any user participation must be fully resourced. The user should be gaining from personal development and helping others, and the service gaining from input and the promotion of its activities to others.

Formal protocols

Written protocols should be utilised where possible and include the following.

- User participation should be written into the service level agreement or contract between the commissioner or funders and the service.

- All services should have a written strategy for user involvement.
- Protocols on how needle exchange is administered, methadone is dispensed, supervised consumption, rights and responsibilities of service users, complaints procedures and how people are treated when waiting should be formally drawn up and disseminated to patients.

Regular feedback

The service user is in the perfect position to comment on the accessibility, availability, care co-ordination, outcome and quality of their treatment. User involvement in services is often limited to feedback on the services they have accessed. This could take the form of satisfaction questionnaires, focus groups or any other method of collating user views. These results can be skewed by participants not wanting to openly criticise the service and it does not reach those not accessing services.

Under-represented groups should be positively targeted. There is a role for user groups or representatives in accessing hard to reach groups such as sexworkers, BME groups, stimulant users, etc. Informal peer networks can identify unmet need and gain privileged access to drug using populations.

- Ensure that user feedback mechanisms are effective.
- Evaluation questionnaires should be made available and anonymous.
- Utilise as many different feedback mechanisms as possible to gain a full picture of your service.

Training and personal development

Training and personal development is imperative to non-tokenistic user involvement. Expertise can be shared between professionals and users.

- Staff could offer in-house training sessions to users.
- Invite service user representatives to staff training sessions.
- Include service users, where practical, in team meetings.
- Service users could offer training to staff.

If users are to be involved in longer term projects they will have to be fully resourced.

- Administrative support and/or access to computers may be necessary.
- Service users should be promptly reimbursed for out-of-pocket expenses.
- Childcare provision should be offered.
- A realistic project timescale should be agreed.

Suggestions for user involvement
- Giving input to team meetings.
- Being an 'information buddy' to new workers to the field during induction.
- Identifying information needs and developing resources and literature.
- Reviewing policies and procedures.

- Representing service users on management committees and/or Board level meetings.
- Providing training to professionals.
- Current and ex-users could be employed in paid and unpaid positions.
- Conducting independent research or being respondents.
- Helping to identify unmet need by gaining privileged access to under-represented groups.
- Encouraging peers to take up vaccinations against bloodborne viruses.
- Delivering peer education to service users.
- Consulting with service users on relevant issues.
- Providing feedback on good and bad practice.
- Passing on good information (e.g. harm reduction techniques) through peer networks.
- Being involved in recruitment processes, e.g. sitting on interview panels.
- Developing user-focused guidelines.
- Evaluating the service and identifying areas for change.
- Informing others of user involvement mechanisms.
- Conducting needs assessment exercises projects and inputting changes.
- Co-ordinating the dissemination of warning messages regarding the circulation of contaminated drugs.

Box 3.11 Summary

- Services should include users in their operations and inclusion protocols should be drawn up.
- Users will need to be supported, informed and fully resourced.
- Users should gain personal development from involvement.

Patient consultation in strategic decision making

User involvement in strategy and policy making will ensure that the rights of the individual and needs of users are regarded as integral to the treatment system as a whole.

The NTA is committed to user involvement in all aspects of its business. It has user and carer representation on its Board, utilises an 'expert group' to inform strategy and policy and is developing a permanent advisory group constituted of users and carer representatives. National Treatment Agency guidance states that drug user views should be incorporated into policy making at a national level, and locally, into agencies and DATs.

Drug action teams (are required to evidence user involvement locally by ensuring users play a primary role in the consultation process to inform annual treatment plans. Drug action teams should be including user involvement processes in all service level agreements and in the reviewing process. Drug action teams should also support local user groups and user representation.

User groups can present a case for change in service delivery, pressurise decision makers to take account of user views and represent users in a whole raft of related issues.

Box 3.12 Summary

- Users are involved in policy making and strategic planning of drug treatment.
- Users should be fully involved in D(A)AT treatment planning processes.
- User representation can effect change.

Summary

Effective user involvement leads to improved treatment for, and of, drug users. Ensuring a two-way communication flow between users and services will provide transparency and lead to flexible and appropriate working practices. Consumer involvement makes good business sense, and should be a key element of monitoring and evaluating service delivery. The benefits of meaningful user involvement in drug treatment discourse can be felt by users, practitioners, drug services, commissioners, policy makers and the wider community.

National drug user organisations

Black Poppy – is a national user-led magazine aimed at users. Services can purchase copies and current and ex-users can order them free of charge. www.blackpoppy.org.uk

The Alliance (formerly The Methadone Alliance) – offers and promotes peer advocacy, training and support to user groups and representatives. The organisation offers a national helpline and has local advocates in many areas. The Alliance inputs to policy making, the evidence base for prescribing and promotes user involvement in all its work. www.m-alliance.org.uk

The Development Agency (formerly the National Drug Users Development Agency) – is a membership organisation that provides support, training, advice and information to new and existing user groups. Tel: 020 8986 5475.

UKHRA coalition – The United Kingdom Harm Reduction Alliance is a campaigning coalition of drug users, health and social care workers, criminal justice workers and educationalists that aims to put public health and human rights at the centre of drug treatment and service provision for drug users. www.ukhra.org.uk

References

1   Farrell C (2004) *Patient and Public Involvement in Health: the evidence for policy implementation*. Department of Health, London.

2 Drug Strategy Directorate (2002) *Updated Drug Strategy*. HMSO, London.

3 Nelles B (2004) *Users Leading Change*. Proceedings of the 2nd National Drug Treatment Conference, 4–5 March, 2004. London.

4 Department of Health (2000) *The NHS Plan: a plan for investment, a plan for reform*. HMSO, London.

5 NTA and Drugscope (2003) *Enhancing Drug Services*. Drugscope Publications, London.

6 Shiner M (2000) *Doing It for Themselves: an evaluation of peer approaches to drug prevention*. HMSO, London.

7 McDermott P (2003) *Out-patient Treatment for Heroin Addiction: a service-users' guide to rights and responsibilities*. Lifeline Publications, Manchester.

8 National Treatment Agency (2002) *Models of Care for Treatment of Adult Drug Misusers*. National Treatment Agency, London.

9 Task Force to Review Services for Drug Misusers (1996) *Report of an Independent Review of Drug Treatment Services in England*. Department of Health, London.

10 Department of Health (1997) *Purchasing Effective Treatment and Care for Drug Misusers: guidance for health authorities and social services departments*. Department of Health, London.

11 SCODA (1997) *Enhancing Drug Services*. SCODA, London.

12 SCODA (1997) *Getting Drug Users Involved: good practice in local treatment and planning*. SCODA, London.

13 Fleming P (2001) *The Role of Treatment Services in Motivating and Deterring Treatment Entry*. Wells Healthcare Communications Ltd, Kent.

14 Gossop M (2003) *NTORS: Choose Maintenance or Detoxification, not 'Reduction'*. Network Newsletter No. 5. SMMGP, London.

CHAPTER 4

The role of the practice nurse in substance misuse treatments

Tracey Campbell and *Jane Gray*

Introduction

Nurses working in general practice settings are ideally placed to engage with clients who have substance misuse issues, as often they are the first point of contact that clients have in primary care. Working as a primary care nurse with clients with drug dependency issues can be a challenging yet often rewarding experience. Clients with drug dependence often present with complex and multiple health needs and managing these requires the nurse to use problem-solving skills to identify creative solutions to difficult problems. Whilst health promotion and education should always be individualised to clients needs, this is especially important with those who have drug dependency issues. This chapter provides information, guidance and advice for primary care nurses working with clients who have drug dependence.

Common presentations of health problems

Clients with an addiction may present with a variety of health problems and the assessment and management should reflect the client's priorities. Whilst by no means exhaustive, this chapter focuses more deeply on the following selection of common health issues specific to clients with drug dependence which primary care nurses may appropriately address.

- Malnutrition.
- Women's health and screening issues.
- Sexual health and contraception.
- Issues associated with addiction and harm reduction advice.

In 1998 the *Big Issue* of the North undertook a health needs survey of vendors in Leeds, Manchester and Liverpool looking at common health problems reported by *Big Issue* street vendors.[1] The results are shown in Box 4.1. They also considered addiction issues, sexual practices and access to primary and secondary care services.

Box 4.1   Sample of health needs

Addiction
   Alcohol
   Drug
Minor ailments
   Minor injuries
   Wound care
   Foot care
   Head lice
   Dermatology
   Dental
Chronic disease management
   Coronary heart disease (CHD)
   Asthma
   Diabetes
   Hepatitis and HIV
Men's health
   Sexual health/contraception
   Safety
   Testicular self-examination
   Prostate awareness

Mental health
   Anxiety
   Depression
   Loneliness
   Isolation
   Suicide
   Self-harm
   Paranoia
   Personality disorder
   Psychosis
   Schizophrenia
Sexual health
   Screening
   Condom distribution
Women's health
   Sexual health/contraception
   Safety
   Pregnancy
   Breast awareness
   Cervical cytology

Curran and Flannigan suggest that drug-using clients give low priority to their health needs due to having low self-esteem, poor perception of health needs and the difficulties experienced when trying to access services. They state, 'Personal autonomy and responsibility for health appears to need to be nurtured and actively encouraged within this population. It is suggested that empowerment of individuals in this way may increase self-esteem and raise their perception of health and what they as individuals can do to enhance it.'[2] Primary care nurses can do much to empower clients and interest them in their health, by adopting a non-judgemental approach and offering flexible, accessible and appropriate services which reflect their needs.

Malnutrition

A variety of studies of homeless populations, which included drug users, identified that both homeless populations and drug users have a lower body mass index (BMI) score in comparison to that of the general population.[3–5] Whilst obesity is often an issue with the general population who may present in primary care, drug users in contrast may present with signs of multiple malnutrition. Primary care nurses need to be mindful of this common problem. Box 4.2 gives BMI categories and identifies the three types of malnutrition associated with drug users.[6]

Box 4.2   BMI categories and drug-user malnutrition types

BMI categories:
- <19 underweight
- 20–25 desirably healthy
- 26–30 overweight
- >30 obese

Three malnutrition types:
1 Micronutrient deficiency
2 Kwashiorkor-type malnutrition (protein)
3 Marasmus malnutrition (fat)

The management of poor nutrition within the drug using population is often addressed by introducing supplementary nutritional feeds. Prescribing guidelines recommend these are only introduced to clients with a BMI of <19 and the intention is for short-term use.

However, nurses should continue to discuss nutritional management with clients with a BMI >19 as they will still be at risk of malnutrition and micro-nutrient deficiency.

Noble and McCombie suggest that routine use of supplement nutrition should be discouraged and found injecting drug users reduced their intake of solid food whilst on supplements due to having unrealistic expectations of weight gain.[7] They also developed flavour fatigue and thus discontinued them. In conclusion they state that dietary advice and counselling to encourage increased solid food intake have improved results within these clients. The authors advise that nutritional advice should include practical solutions within a low budget and take into account social factors. However Langnase and Muller, Darmon *et al.* and Islam *et al.* suggest that when managing malnutrition and weight gain a combination of supplements and health education is essential.[3–5]

Community dieticians can advise on appropriate nutrition and eating plans, particularly on a small budget and with poor facilities and are a good source to utilise. Primary care nurses can offer general advice on healthy eating regimes and encourage regular intake of small frequent meals as drug users may be chaotic and 'forget' to eat.

When discussing nutritional health education the following resources available to these clients and their practical skills should be taken into account:

- budgeting skills
- access to cooking and storage facilities
- shopping and cooking skills
- income
- motivation and self-esteem to go shopping
- how to access services that provide food.

Rollins promotes the use of screening tools by healthcare professionals in the assessment of malnutrition and expresses the view that nutritional screening is a key part of the clinical governance agenda as poor nutrition has serious physical and psychosocial consequences.[8] Screening tools aid the recording of information and give a qualitative measure of nutritional risk rather than a subjective assessment, which can be repeated in the evaluation process.[6] The use of screening tools with drug using clients needs to be quick and simple but effective. There are a variety of tools available, for example the MUST tool available on the website www.bapen.org.uk.

Women's health

Women with dependency issues historically have a low uptake of primary health-care services particularly screening and health promotion/prevention activities. This may be for a variety of reasons, such as:

- poor perception of health needs and health beliefs
- negative past experiences of accessing primary or secondary services
- marginalisation, discrimination or isolation experiences
- controlling relationship or domestic violence
- perceived belief or reprisal in relation to child care or fear of social services involvement due to drug use.

Providing a 'women only' environment or clinic session at your practice staffed by female staff and/or introducing alternative therapies for women to engage with to nurture a trusting relationship with the team were found to be valuable in a general practice setting. A pilot of offering massage and aromatherapy at the NFA Health Team in Leeds over a three month period was a positive experience for both the women accessing the clinic and the nursing team, and aromatherapy and acupuncture have evaluated well for both men and women drug using clients in Leicestershire.

Cervical screening

There are around 3500 new cases of cervical cancer and approximately 1200 deaths from the disease annually in the UK. Since 1988 the NHS has provided a national cervical screening programme with the overall aim of reducing the morbidity and mortality associated with cervical cancer. Experts predict that around 3900 cases of cervical cancer are prevented each year.[9]

A variety of health and social factors may contribute to the increased risk of women developing cervical cancer and are shown in the list. Nurses gaining a history from their clients are in an ideal position to identify these risk factors.[10,11]

- Women in a low socio-economic class, particularly IV and V.
- Early first intercourse.
- Multiple sexual partners and partners who have had multiple sexual partners.
- Non-use of barrier contraception.
- Early first pregnancy, which increases with subsequent pregnancies.

- Smoking.
- Human papilloma virus (DNA types 16 and 18).

Studies have shown that women with addiction may fulfil some or many of the above risk factors coupled with poor engagement of primary care services and women's perception of health screening may be of a low priority.[12,13] Nurses offering cervical screening on an opportunistic basis or when a good relationship has been established may significantly improve uptake as was the experience of the Leicester Homeless Primary Healthcare Service where uptake increased from 50% in 2001 to 80% in 2004 (author's audit data). Factors to take into account when offering screening are:

- women's understanding of the screening process
- system in place which ensures women receive their results from a central service or from the practice and that results are not delayed
- previous sexual abuse or assault history may make women reluctant to undergo intimate procedures and sensitivity is needed
- women's perception of health and risk
- relationship between nurse and client.

Sexual health and contraception

Sexual health and contraception are important issues to address with drug users as often these aspects of health assume a low priority with clients who may be undertaking risky behaviour. With women, these issues can be addressed and included when discussing smears and women may opt for routine swab taking during a smear to screen for infections. It is important to remember that these are issues that should be raised with male clients too. Nurses can offer:

- sexually transmitted infection (STI) screening (including *Chlamydia*) and provision of local centre details for sexual health and family planning services
- supplies of condoms and lubrication
- contraceptive advice and provision of methods
- information and cards with contact details and information of local inter-agency services for:
  - victims of rape or assault
  - those fleeing domestic violence
  - those in need of counselling, support or housing advice
- pregnancy testing, advice and referral to specialist services
- if men or women are working in the sex industry, be aware of local support networks and signpost to these local projects, which provide a sexual health and advocacy service.

When considering contraceptive options take into account:

- concordance with method, for example the taking of a pill each day within time limits
- encourage use of condoms with all methods of contraception to prevent STIs

- use of placebo contraceptive samples when discussing options to aid client's visualisation of the methods.

Bloodborne viruses – prevalence and information

Globally hepatitis B affects 30% of the world's population and one per 1000 of the UK population and hepatitis C affects 3% of the world's population and 600 000 of the UK population. Human immunodeficiency virus (HIV), although less common is rising rapidly and with a global population exceeding 60 billion, approximately 40 million people are infected with HIV; approximately 3000 or 0.3% are in Western Europe.

Hepatitis is defined as inflammation of the liver and although viral infection (A–G) is the most common cause within the drug using population, hepatitis can also occur through bacterial infection, toxins, alcohol or drug use and trauma. Clients may present with:

- flu-like symptoms
- fatigue
- loss of appetite
- jaundice
- nausea and vomiting
- abdominal pain
- cognitive impairments.

Clients may have no symptoms or a combination of the above either constantly or intermittently. If in doubt, a review by a medical practitioner is advisable for prompt assessment, diagnosis, access to treatment and prevention of transmission to others. Clients will require admission to hospital and the public health team at the Health Protection Agency (HPA) must also be notified.

Screening and immunisation

Screening

When offering a screening service for drug users it is valuable to offer a pre- and post-test discussion session with the client at the time of taking the blood sample and when giving the results. Nurses should be aware that the recall of information given to clients declines quickly with an estimated retention of only one third of the information given; this decreases with the increase of information given. Local research of a study of 17 homeless drug users interviewed after giving a positive hepatitis result showed that clients continued to need support or reiteration of information up to several years after diagnosis and they expressed that the diagnosis had a lasting emotional impact on them.[14]

Nurses offering a screening service should be familiar with local secondary care services policies or formulate working partnerships with the infectious diseases, hepatology and genito-urinary medicine (GUM) unit nurse specialists for information and support. This is valuable when developing referral pathways for drug users.

Pre-test discussion
- What you are screening for – hepatitis B, C and HIV.
- What the client's risk factors are.
- Explain about the window period of the viruses.
- Prepare the client for a negative and positive test at this stage.
- Confidentiality.
- Arrange for the client to return for a post-test discussion when receiving the results.
- Discuss legal issues of record keeping and medical notes so the client is aware of potential impact of mortgage or insurance company's policies.
- Harm reduction opportunity.

Post-test discussion
Negative result
- Advise the client to repeat the screening test in three and six months to allow for the window period where a false-negative may occur whilst the disease is incubating.
- Opportunity to discuss harm reduction.

Positive result
- To confirm continued infection of the virus a PCR or RNA blood sample must be sent at this stage:
  – positive PCR: discussion or referral to secondary care is next stage
  – negative PCR: repeat in six months – after two negative PCR results the client can be informed they have cleared the virus.
- Liver function test (LFT) clotted blood sample sent to the chemical pathology laboratory.
- Discuss referral to secondary care to the infectious diseases unit or gastro-enterology/hepatology department for treatment of the virus and explain possible further investigations and treatment processes.
- Harm reduction opportunity to prevent transmission of virus.
- Contact tracing can be undertaken independently or jointly with the public health team at the Health Protection Agency if necessary.
- Support services available locally.

A leaflet should be given to the client at pre- and post-test discussion; leaflets are available through some practices and community drug teams. Alternatively, it may be appropriate to produce a practice leaflet specific to your policies or protocols about pre- and post-test discussions.

Blood samples for screening
A clotted sample of blood is sent to the virology department of the pathology laboratory to test for bloodborne virus status. The initial test is an antibody test for hepatitis B, C and HIV. 'Antigen positive' means there is active virus and the client is infectious. 'Antibody positive' means that antibody has been produced to defend against a virus the client has had contact with (surface antibody levels are present after immunisation). A polymerase chain reaction (PCR) indicates continued reproduction of the virus.

Pre-treatment investigation or interventions

Lifestyle changes
- Harm reduction
- Healthy diet
- Rest
- Reduction or abstinence of alcohol
- Methadone maintenance or detoxification from drugs
- Sexual health information.

Investigations
- Full blood screening as indicated or requested by the hepatology department
- Liver biopsy
- Liver ultrasound.

Treatment
Current practice in the treatment of hepatitis C is to use pegalated interferon and ribavirin combination therapy. Therapy may be for a period of six or 12 months. Interferons are proteins, which naturally occur as part of the defence mechanism and are produced in response to infection; they interfere with virus replication. Ribavirin is an antiviral drug: antiviral drugs either prevent the virus from reproducing or destroy the virus thus clearing the viral infection. Ribavirin is the recommended drug for the treatment of hepatitis C.

Hepatitis B: current guidelines for the treatment of hepatitis B are to treat with interferon alpha or lamivudine, a nucleoside analogue that is a potent inhibitor of the viral DNA replication.

Human immunodeficiency virus (HIV): a combination of treatment regimes are offered to patients with HIV. For further information, contact your local treatment centre or the Terence Higgins Trust.

Immunisations

Hepatitis A and B immunisation should be offered to the client at the earliest opportunity and the immunisation of drug users must never be postponed whilst waiting for blood results for bloodborne viruses, as no harm will come to them even if they prove to be positive to hepatitis B, C or HIV. Administration of vaccines by nurses is facilitated by working to Patient Group Directions from the employing PCT. Extended nurse prescribers can prescribe and administer vaccines in their own right. Hepatitis A and B vaccines can be administered as single or combined antigens. Box 4.3 gives guidance on the regimes.

Box 4.3   Immunisation regimes

Hepatitis A vaccine:
Initial dose then booster dose at six to 12 months. With booster expect a ten year protection period.

Hepatitis B vaccine:
Standard schedule: Initial dose, second dose at one month and third at six months – thus zero, one, six month intervals.

Rapid schedule: Initial dose, second dose at one month and third dose at two months and fourth completing dose at 12 months – thus zero, one, two, 12 month intervals.

Exceptional schedule: Initial dose, second dose at seven days, third dose at 21 days and fourth completing dose at 12 months – thus zero, seven, 21 day and 12 month intervals.

Note: exceptional schedule is not licensed for <18 years of age.
Second and third doses are calculated from initial dose.
Compliance with regime may alter per client. If second dose is missed within one year, give second dose then third dose three months after (Engerix Vaccine policy from GlaxoSmithKline).

Hepatitis A, B combined vaccine:
Standard schedule: Initial dose, second dose at one month and third dose at six months – thus zero, one, six month intervals.

Rapid schedule: Initial dose, second dose at seven days, third dose at 21 days and fourth completing dose at 12 months – thus 0, 7, 21 days and 12 months.

Note: A blood test may be taken at eight weeks post third vaccine for sero-conversion status. Approximately 2% of those having the vaccine may not sero-convert and may need to complete a second course of the vaccine.

A study over a two-year period of completion of hepatitis vaccination in a drug using population showed that compliance to the standard regime was low, most clients only completing the first or second dose.[15] The introduction of the exceptional schedule with this client group showed an increase of completion rates. This regime was piloted as part of the outreach immunisation service for drug users citywide and in comparison to outreach services offering the standard schedule, showed a higher completion rate using the exceptional schedule. Hewett *et al.* mirrors these findings and reports a 100% increase in completed hepatitis vaccination courses by switching from a standard to rapid schedule.[16] Therefore, the authors recommend that the four dose exceptional schedule is adopted when vaccinating this client group.

Tetanus immunisation is also an important consideration for injecting drug users, particularly in response to a recent national outbreak of heroin infected with *Clostridium tetani* (July 2003–July 2004). Within the 12-month time frame 22 cases were identified nationally with pockets in the North West and Midland areas of the UK. The usual annual background rate for the whole of the UK is usually five to ten cases. All individuals were injecting drug users. The Joint Committee for Vaccines and Immunisations (JCVI) has recommended that tetanus vaccination status is checked with injecting drug users and they are offered vaccines as appropriate. However, as single antigen tetanus vaccine is no longer available a combination of tetanus toxoid (40 iu) and diphtheria (4 iu) should be given as per national guidance. If a client has not received a primary course (five doses in their lifetime) this must be given. Box 4.4 gives guidance on the regimes.

Box 4.4   Immunisation regimes

Tetanus/diphtheria:
Primary schedule: Initial dose, second dose at one month and third at two months, then booster at 10 years and 20 years – thus zero, one month, two month, 10 year and 20 year intervals.

Boosters: After primary schedule give a single booster dose every 10 years whilst client is continuing to inject street drugs.

Addiction

When a new client registers at the practice there is an ideal opportunity to take an initial history or assessment of their health needs and through this process addiction issues may come to light. The use of templates when using an electronic record system may be of value as prompts may be included in the new patient registration screen. For practices where this system is not available the following questions may be a useful guide when a dependency issue has been raised. The questions may also be adapted in the use of assessment of alcohol addiction.

What is the client's drug of choice?
• The client may either have one drug of choice or be a poly (many) drugs user. Ask the series of questions for each drug being used. For drugs no longer used establish when the client last used the drug.

When did the client first start using the drug?
• May give a picture of the drug use history of the client.

How much drug of choice per day in pounds is used?
• The measurement of monetary pounds is used as it is often easier for the nurse and client to visualise the amount of drug being taken rather than using grams, which may be interpreted differently by each party. In general, although this may change with region, heroin comes in bags of £10 or £15.
• The quality of the drug may change regionally or with supplies of the drug in the community. Knowing the amount of drug a client is using is essential to the assessment of commencing an opiate detoxification regime.
• You may wish to record how often they are using the drug daily.

How is the client administering the drug?
• Establish how the client is administering the drug, for example snorting, injecting, smoking.

Last detoxification: date, how long were they drug free, what support did the client receive?
• May give an indication of what worked well for the client and things that have not been successful.
• May influence the decision making process when choosing the right detoxification regime.

Box 4.5   Drug related illness

- DVT
- Abscess
- Fibrosis
- Overdose
- Hepatitis B and/or C
- HIV
- Cellulitis
- Septicaemia
- Streptococcal infection
- Ulcer
- Gangrene
- Endocarditis

Any current drug related illness?
- Box 4.5 lists drug related illness for common presentations.

Client's expectations of current drug use?
- Establish if the client is requesting a referral for a detoxification programme or is planning to continue their drug use.
- If referring for detoxification you may wish to ascertain:
  - if they have considered what detoxification regime they would like to try
  - what social support they have and residency stability.
- If no detoxification at this time this may be an opportunity for a harm reduction intervention.

Additional information?
- Hepatitis and HIV screening history.
- Hepatitis B or A/B immunisation history.
- Is the client currently or previously working with any local drug projects or needle exchange projects? If not you may wish to signpost the client to local resources.

Referral to drug detoxification?
- Awareness of local service providers.
- Local detoxification policy.
- Send a plain urine sample (taken on the premises) for an opiate drug screen to the chemical pathology department of the pathology laboratory.

Table 4.1 provides a summary of drug groups. Box 4.6 lists injecting equipment.

Table 4.1 Drug group summary

Drug group	Example	Street name	Administration route
Hallucinogens	Cannabis	Spliff	Smoked mixed with tobacco or in a pipe
	Amphetamine	E's (ecstasy)	Swallowed as pills or capsules
Uppers	Cocaine/crack	Charlie/rocks	Snorted or injected. Freebase is smoked
Downers	Benzodiazepines	Sleepers	Swallowed as pills or capsules
	Solvents and gases		Vapours inhaled through nose or mouth
Opiates	Heroin	Smack/gear	Smoked or injected
Opioids	Methadone		Liquid form
	Buprenorphine	Jellies	swallowed or injected

Box 4.6   Injecting paraphernalia

Syringes
Needles
Spoons or other cooking-up containers
Water
Water containers
Alcohol swabs
Filters
Preparation surface
Acidifiers
Tourniquet
Lighters

Crack pipes
Straws for snorting

Harm reduction

Harm reduction is the process of providing information and guidance, which enables clients to make informed choices about their health and in this context their drug use practices. Abstaining from drugs may be a long-term plan or aim for clients but in the quest to achieve this clients need to be aware of the risks to their health associated with the administration of street drugs, and practical messages to reduce these risks must be given and reinforced at each contact.

Table 4.2   Harm reduction measures in drug administration routes

Least harm	Harmful	Avoid	Alternatives
Arms	Breasts (fragile veins – risk of infection)	Neck (risk of hitting major artery or nerves)	'Up ya bum' (administration of heroin through absorption in anal canal)
Hands (inject slowly – fragile veins)	Feet (fragile veins – painful)	Groin (risk of hitting artery or nerves. High risk of infection and DVT)	Smoking (much safer way to take substances)
Back of the leg (inject slowly)	Intramuscular injection (not a long-term option)	Penis (risk of infections and painful erections)	Sniffing
Subcutaneous injecting (skin popping – chance of infection due to lack of oxygen)			Swallowing (allow time for effects to take place before topping up)

- Rather than a long list of what not to do, discuss the process of transmission to ascertain understanding and increased knowledge of the risks of cross-infection.[17]
- Training is available for nurses and workers with this client group.
- Provide information of local needle exchange and drug projects.

Tables 4.2 and 4.3 suggest practical messages that may be used with clients.

Deep vein thrombosis (DVT)

There is an increasing incidence of clients injecting heroin and crack into femoral veins in the groin.

This has resulted in an increase in presentation to primary and secondary care services with health related problems associated with groin injecting, in particular abscesses and infections and worryingly DVT, which has resulted in pulmonary embolism (PE).

As part of the harm reduction process, raising awareness of the problems of groin injecting and discussing alternative sites or methods of administration is vital.

Deep vein thrombosis leaflets for professionals and drug users are available from many health promotion resources departments, community drug services and in some general practices.

Table 4.3 Harm reduction measures in drug use

Safer injecting	Preventing initiation into injecting	Hepatitis B vaccination	Overdose prevention and response	Smoking	Sharing and lending
Always inject towards the heart. Rotate veins	Messages to injectors	Hepatitis B is carried in blood, vaginal fluid, semen, small amounts in urine and saliva	If someone overdoses don't assume they'll come round	Smoking is a much safer alternative to injecting	Sharing or lending injecting equipment risks transmission of bloodborne viruses
Choose the smallest possible needle	Don't talk about injecting to non-injectors	It can be passed in blood and sexual fluids	Don't panic	It reduces the risk of catching bloodborne viruses such as HIV and hepatitis B/C	Do not share or lend any injecting equipment
Try to keep everything clean	Don't inject in front of non-injectors	You can be vaccinated	Put them in the recovery position	It reduces chances of getting injecting injuries	This includes needles, filters, spoons, water, etc.
Inject at a shallow angle	Don't give people their first hit	Ask your doctor	Dial 999	There is less risk of overdose	Front- or back-loading also risks infection
Loosen tourniquet before injecting		There is NO vaccination for hepatitis C	Stay with them until an ambulance arrives		
INJECT SLOWLY			Police are usually not called to overdoses		
Straight after injecting apply pressure to site			Ask your drug service about local policies		

Tables 4.2 and 4.3: Part of DVT Leeds training package. Leeds DAT, NE-PCT and NFT Team.

Health promotion and health education

Health promotion can be defined as 'any planned measure which promotes health or prevents disease, disability and premature death' (education model), and to 'provide information and create empowerment' (empowerment model).

Also, 'The person will be able to make informed choices with regard to prevention of ill health; changes of behaviour; use of appropriate services and have an awareness of environmental and social factors influencing health' (preventative medical model).[18]

SMART

The measures should be:

- **S**pecific
- **M**easurable
- **A**chievable
- **R**ealistic
- **T**imed.

Factors that affect the assessment process and health promotion are as follows.

- Maslow's hierarchy of need.
- Influence of alcohol and drugs.
- Mental health status.
- Violence and aggression.
- Pre-conceived experience and ideas.
- Beliefs and attitudes.

How to implement health promotion in addiction[19]

- One-to-one
- Displays
- Leaflets
- Pictorial
- Practical
- Opportunistic
- Five-minute interaction
- Flexibility
- Realistic
- Adapt health promotion to lifestyle and resources available to client
- Prioritise your harm reduction intervention
- Listen to your patient
- Keep messages simple and to a minimum
- Use appropriate language
- Review and reiterate
- The process of change model (*see* Figure 4.1).

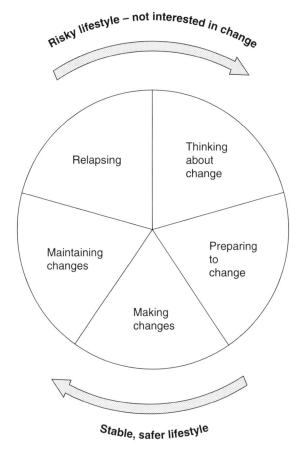

Figure 4.1 The addiction cycle.

References

1 Big Issue of the North (1998) *A Primary Health Care Study of Vendors of the 'Big Issue' of the North.* Manchester.
2 Curran CI and Flanningan CE (1997) *Belfast's single homeless health care project.* THS quality in health in Northern Ireland. Cited in *Big Issue of the North.*
3 Langnase K and Muller MJ (2001) Nutrition and health in an adult homeless population in Germany. *Public Health Nutrition.* **4**(3): 805–11.
4 Darmon N, Coupel J, Deheeger M *et al.* (2001) Dietary inadequacies observed in homeless men visiting an emergency night shelter in Paris. *Public Health Nutrition.* **4**(2): 155–61.
5 Islam SKN, Hossain KJ, Ahmed A *et al.* (2002) Nutritional status of drug addicts undergoing detoxification: prevalence of malnutrition and influence of illicit drugs and life style. *British Journal of Nutrition.* **88**(5): 507–13.
6 McClaren S (1998) Nutritional screening and assessment. *Nursing Standard.* **12**(48): 26–9.

7   Noble C and McCombie L (1997) Nutritional considerations in intravenous drug misusers: a review of the literature and current issues for dietitians. *Journal of Human Nutrition and Dietetics.* **10**: 181–91.

8   Rollins H (2002) Implementing a screening programme. *Primary Health Care.* **12**(1): 38–9.

9   Department of Health (1999) *Report on Cervical Screening Programme.* Government Response to Public Accounts Committee. Reference Number: 1999/0153. Department of Health, London.

10   Neilson A and Jones R (1998) Women's lay knowledge of cervical cancer/screening: accounting for non-attenders at cervical screening clinics. *Journal of Advanced Nursing.* **28**(3): 571–5.

11   Sutherland C (2001) *Women's Health: a handbook for nurses.* Churchill Livingstone, London.

12   Wright N (1999) *Homelessness: a primary care response.* Royal College of General Practitioners, London.

13   Patnick J (1999) *Cervical Screening: a pocket guide.* National Health Service Cervical Screening Programme, Sheffield.

14   Tompkins CNE, Wright NMJ and Jones L (2004) 'It's always at the back of your mind.' The Impact of a Positive Hepatitis C Diagnosis on Homeless Injecting Drug Users. Submitted for publication to *British Journal of General Practice.*

15   Wright NMJ, Campbell TL and Tompkins CNE (2002) A comparison of conventional and accelerated hepatitis B immunisation schedules for homeless drug users. *Communicable Disease and Public Health.* **5**(4): 324–6.

16   Hewett N, Gray J, Hiley A *et al.* (2003) *Annual Report of the Leicester Homeless Primary Healthcare Service.* April 2002 – March 2003. Leicestershire Partnership NHS Trust, Leicestershire.

17   Derricott J, Preston A and Hunt N (1999) *The Safer Injecting Brief: an easy to use comprehensive reference guide to promoting safer injecting.* HIT Publications.

18   www.healthpromotionagency.org.uk

19   Prochaska J and DiClemente C (1983) Stages and process of self change. *Journal of Consulting and Clinical Psychology.* **51**: 390–5.

CHAPTER 5

Primary care nursing and alcohol: a new way forward?

Richard Bryant-Jefferies

Introduction

This chapter gives a brief overview of the *Alcohol Harm Reduction Strategy for England*.[1] The Strategy highlights many valid areas to address, and there is no new money outlined for already often over-stretched alcohol services. The chapter focuses specifically on what the Strategy suggests with regard to improving information flow, and the identification and treatment of alcohol misuse.

'Brief interventions' are also described; already a key element of the primary healthcare response to identifying and responding to patients with alcohol problems. Evidence for brief interventions is highlighted and the 'cycle of change' model which provides a theoretical framework for this work is outlined.

National Alcohol Strategy

The scale of the impact of alcohol use on primary healthcare provision is enormous. With alcohol related deaths running at around 22 000 each year in Great Britain (approximately one death every 24 minutes),[1] (p. 7) and over 30 000 hospital admissions each year for alcohol dependence syndrome (many more admissions will be the result of other alcohol related problems including accidents and violence), the need for credible healthcare responses is vital.

The Executive Summary of the Strategy reports: 'The Strategy Unit's interim analysis estimated that alcohol misuse is now costing around £20 billion a year. This is made up of alcohol related health disorders and disease, crime and anti-social behaviour, loss of productivity in the workplace, and problems for those who misuse alcohol and their families, including domestic violence.' (*See* Box 5.1.)

Box 5.1   The annual 'cost' of alcohol misuse[1]

- 1.2 million violent incidents (around half of all violent crime)
- 360 000 incidents of domestic violence (around a third of all domestic violence) linked to alcohol misuse

Continued

- increased antisocial behaviour and fear of crime – 61% of the population perceive alcohol related violence as worsening
- expenditure of £95 million on specialist alcohol treatment
- over 30 000 hospital admissions for alcohol dependence syndrome
- up to 22 000 premature deaths per annum
- at peak times, up to 70% of all admissions to A&E
- up to 1000 suicides
- up to 17 million working days lost through alcohol related absence
- between 780 000 and 1.3 million children affected by parental alcohol problems
- increased divorce – marriages where there are alcohol problems are twice as likely to end in divorce

The Strategy highlights the following drinking patterns that are most likely to increase the risk of harm.

Binge-drinkers: 'those who drink to get drunk and are likely to be aged under 25'.[1] (p. 7) As it is difficult to ascertain numbers of people who go out to get drunk, the Strategy used the numbers of those 'who drank above double the recommended daily guidelines on at least one occasion in the last week'. 'Using this as a measure of "binge" drinking we estimate that around 5.9 million adults drink above this level. Within this group there will be many who are regularly drinking far more than twice the recommended daily amount. Many others will do so only rarely.'[1] (p. 15)

'Binge-drinkers are ... more likely to be men, although women's drinking has been rising fast over the last ten years. Binge drinkers are at increased risk of accidents and alcohol poisoning. Men in particular are more likely both to be a victim of violence and to commit violent offences. There can also be a greater risk of sexual assault. The impacts on society are visible in, for example, high levels of attendance at A&E related to alcohol.'[1] (p. 7)

Chronic drinkers: 'those who are drinking large amounts regularly. Around a quarter of the population drink above the former weekly guidelines of 14 units for women and 21 units for men; with 6.4 million drinking above the harmful limits of 35 units per week for women and 50 units a week for men; and a further 1.8 million, two-thirds of them men, drink above these levels.'[1] (p. 15) 'These drinkers are more likely to be aged over 30 and around two-thirds are men. They are at increased risk of a variety of health harms such as cirrhosis (which has nearly doubled in the last ten years), cancer, haemorrhagic stroke, premature death and suicide. They are also more likely to commit the offences of domestic violence and drink-driving.'[1] (p. 7)

The importance and role of partnership working is stressed – between the Government, alcohol producers and retailers, health and police services as well as individuals and communities. At a national level 'a social responsibility charter for drinks producers, will strongly encourage drinks companies to:

- pledge not to manufacture products irresponsibly – for example, no products that appeal to under-age drinkers or that encourage people to drink well over recommended limits

- ensure that advertising does not promote or condone irresponsible or excessive drinking
- put the "sensible drinking message" clearly on bottles alongside information about unit content
- move to packaging products in safer materials – for example, alternatives to glass bottles
- make a financial contribution to a fund that pays for new schemes to address alcohol misuse at national and local levels, such as providing information and alternative facilities for young people.'[1] (p. 9)

The Strategy then focuses on the local level where 'there will be a new "code of good conduct" scheme for retailers, pubs and clubs, run locally by a partnership of the drinks industry, police and licensing panels, and led by the local authority. These will ensure that the industry works alongside local communities on issues which really matter, such as under-age drinking and making town centres safer and more welcoming at night. Participation in these schemes will be voluntary'.[1] (p. 9) This is good and whilst the Strategy suggests that the 'success of the voluntary approach will be reviewed early in the next parliament', many will have hoped for something more legislative at this stage. Time will tell as to whether the industry that is profiting from alcohol sales will be prepared to take actions which, in effect, will mean a reduction in alcohol use and therefore profits.

Four key areas of alcohol related harm

The Strategy identifies four key areas or groups of alcohol related harm to be tackled.

1   'Health harms: We calculate the cost of alcohol misuse to the health service to be £1.7 billion per annum. Alcohol misuse is linked to:
- annual expenditure of £95 million on specialist alcohol treatment
- over 30 000 hospital admissions annually for alcohol dependence syndrome
- up to 22 000 premature deaths per annum
- at peak times, up to 70% of all admissions to A&E. (*Interim Analytical Report*, pp. 32–49.)'
In addition, the Chief Medical Officer's *Annual Report for 2001* identified a 'rising trend in deaths from chronic liver disease, with most cases probably being caused by high levels of alcohol consumption'.[1] (pp. 16–17)
2   'Crime and anti-social behaviour harms: We calculate the overall annual cost of crime and anti-social behaviour linked to alcohol misuse to be £7.3 billion. Alcohol misuse shows strong links to violence. 1.2 million violent incidents (around half of all violent crimes) and 360 000 incidents of domestic violence (around a third of these) linked to alcohol misuse. More generally, alcohol misuse is linked to disorder and contributes to driving people's fear of crime; 61% of the population perceive alcohol related violence as worsening. (*Interim Analytical Report*, pp. 50–69.)'[1] (p. 17)
3   'Loss of productivity and profitability: We calculate the overall annual cost of productivity lost as a result of alcohol misuse to be £6.4 billion per annum – up to 17 million working days are lost each year through alcohol

related absence. Alcohol misuse may also affect productivity of workers in their workplace and may result in shorter working lives. (*Interim Analytical Report*, pp. 70–6.)'[1] (p. 17)

4 '**Harms to family and society**: We calculate the cost of the human and emotional impact suffered by victims of alcohol related crime to be £4.7 billion per annum. Between 780 000 and 1.3 million children are affected by parental alcohol problems. Marriages where there are alcohol problems are twice as likely to end in divorce. (*Interim Analytical Report*, pp. 78–86.)'

In addition, 'up to half of rough sleepers have problems with alcohol'.[1] (p. 17)

In order to tackle these areas of alcohol related harm, the Government highlights the following four key aims.[1] (p. 22–3)

1 To improve the information available to individuals and to start the process of change in the culture of drinking to get drunk.
2 To better identify and treat alcohol misuse.
3 To prevent and tackle alcohol related crime and disorder and deliver improved services to victims and witnesses.
4 To work with the industry in tackling the harms caused by alcohol.

Improving information

Drinking is a choice, and for people to be informed about their drinking choices it is important that information is communicated clearly and, where necessary, designed for specific groups of people (young people, women, cultural). The National Alcohol Strategy highlights, in particular, the need for young people to receive 'adequate education on the issue'.[1] There is a need for people to be able to relate the drinks they consume to the information regarding safe drinking. For instance, with varying strengths of alcoholic drinks, the one unit per half pint of beer in the safe drinking message may not relate to the actual strength of a particular person's favourite beer, lager or cider.

Education is not only about amounts consumed. There are also the reasons why people drink, the setting and the context. What role does alcohol have in the family, the community and society at large, and how does a particular culture shape drinking choices and behaviours? What are the individual and collective societal pressures on people to drink? The Strategy indicates that 'the availability of alcohol, its role in our culture and the drinking behaviour by some groups in our society – particularly young people – all affect attitudes, which in turn shape and are shaped by culture. If individuals are to make responsible choices it is just as important to consider how to create social environments which discourage attitudes and behaviours which lead to the risk of harm'.[1] (p. 22)

Information is not only about the effects of alcohol, or the indicators that alcohol use has become problematic and/or that alcohol dependence has developed. It is also about ensuring people know where to get help. Having local resource directories (if only a simple poster with contact information), for instance, available at public places such as libraries and supermarkets, as well as in healthcare, social care, legal and criminal justice settings, offering information as well as indicating where people can seek further help and advice would be valuable. There is also a need for information to reach out to those who do not necessarily go to these places: in cafés, bars and clubs.

'People obtain alcohol related information from five main sources:

- public health information and government campaigns
- information provided by the alcohol industry
- education in schools
- the workplace
- advertising.

Further information may also be provided by friends, families and the wider community.'[1] (p. 27) However, it is clear that information is not reaching people in such a way that they are well enough equipped to make informed choices about their drinking behaviour. The Strategy notes therefore that 'recognition of the Government's "sensible drinking" message is relatively high, with 80% of drinkers having heard of units. But this has little impact on behaviour as only 10% of drinkers check their consumption in units and just 25% know what a "unit" is', and whilst 'school programmes impart information, there is little evidence that they are effective in changing drinking behaviour'.[1] (p. 39)

The Strategy also stresses that the 'levels of awareness of alcohol related problems in the workplace are variable, and responses to our consultation exercise showed increasing concern at how some TV advertising may be condoning (if not encouraging) irresponsible drinking behaviour'.[1] (p. 27) I have to say from my own experience of running alcohol support groups, time and again it is pointed out how difficult it is for drinkers to cope with the constant setting of TV programmes in bars. Whilst these are people already affected by alcohol and seeking to control their use, it indicates that these images do have an effect. For the young person who is developing their own social awareness, and understanding of societal norms, the constant images of alcohol use, and the way it is used, will surely contribute to shaping their own thinking and behaviour. What kind of images do we want to present to young people? What lifestyles do we want to encourage?

It is worth commenting at this point on the use of language. The Strategy talks in terms of 'drinking' alcohol. As someone myself who has worked with people with alcohol problems, and seeing it in the drug treatment context, I tend to think and write in terms of 'using' rather than 'drinking' alcohol. The reality is that consumers of alcohol are using alcohol in order to gain an experience. It may be a sense of being part of a social group, it may be to feel at ease, or reduce stress, a change in mood or perhaps to block out painful and traumatic memories. The reasons are many, but I think it is helpful to think in terms of why people use alcohol, what is their choice about? And, as the strategy points out, for many it is to get drunk although the purpose behind this will vary from individual to individual. To quote from the Strategy: 'It's very important to get drunk. I'm spending money and I want to get drunk, and if I don't it's just a waste of money'. I, too, have heard this said many times. Society seems to be sending clear signals that to get drunk is an important social experience and, indeed, for many it is a sign that a good time is being had. The altering of mood is an important function of drinking alcohol. And this, of course, is an important feature of any choice to use a drug.

In terms of better information and communication the measures within the Strategy aim to:

- 'make the "sensible drinking" message easier to understand and apply
- target campaigns to those most at risk: including binge and chronic drinkers
- share expertise better, both inside and outside Government
- provide better information for consumers, both on products and at the point of sale
- provide alcohol education in schools that can change attitudes and behaviour, as well as raise awareness of alcohol issues
- provide more support and advice for employers
- review the code of practice for TV advertising to ensure that it does not target young drinkers or glamorise irresponsible behaviour.'[1] (p. 39)

Better identification and treatment of alcohol misuse

The Strategy highlights that 'a successful alcohol treatment programme requires:

- the identification and referral of people with alcohol problems
- treatment tailored to differing individual needs and motivations, including support for families where appropriate
- services that are effective in helping vulnerable and at-risk groups.'[1] (p. 39)

It then briefly lists a number of 'problems with the existing identification, referral and treatment services' that need to be addressed:

- 'alcohol problems are often not identified sufficiently early, leading to later financial and human costs
- health service staff have low awareness of alcohol issues
- there is little available information on demand for treatment, the provision of services to meet this demand, or for the current capacity of treatment services
- the structure of alcohol treatment can vary widely, with no clear standards for, or pathways through, treatment
- procedures for referring vulnerable people between alcohol treatment and other services are often unclear.'[1] (p. 39)

The Strategy then continues by indicating that the Government will improve identification and referral processes by:

- 'running pilot programmes to establish whether earlier identification and treatment of those with alcohol problems can improve health, lead to longer term savings, and be embedded into mainstream healthcare provision
- raising health service staff awareness of alcohol misuse issues and improving their ability to deal with them.'

And improve treatment by:

- 'conducting a national audit of alcohol treatment, including the provision of aftercare. This will establish levels of current provision and the extent of unmet demand, to form the basis for improving services

- improving standards of treatment by introducing more co-ordinated arrangements for commissioning and monitoring standards.'[1] (p. 39)

In addition, the Government will 'improve services for vulnerable groups by: commissioning integrated care pathways for the most vulnerable, who often have multiple problems: those with drug problems, mental illness, homeless people and young people.'[1] (p. 39)

In response to the proposal made for improving identification and treatment, Alcohol Concern comments that whilst 'in principle, we welcome the national audit of the capacity of and demand for alcohol service ... we are extremely concerned about the developing crisis in short-term funding. A future audit does nothing for current under-funding and under-capacity. An interim funding initiative for the period until the audit is complete is an absolute necessity.'[2] (p. 2) Also, whilst welcoming the primary care pilots for early interventions as a 'positive development', Alcohol Concern quite rightly points out that it is 'surprised and disappointed at the Government's apparent lack of confidence in the clear existing evidence of the benefits of early interventions.'[2] (p. 2)

'Brief' and 'early' interventions for alcohol misuse

For many people, primary healthcare is the first point of access for help with an alcohol problem. It is estimated that each GP sees 364 heavy drinkers a year.[1] (p. 41) Yet it is estimated that only 'seven or fewer will have their drinking assessed by their doctor'.[2] Of course, it is not only the doctor who may raise alcohol as an issue for discussion with patients; at many GP surgeries the nurse will provide the new patient health check – which includes a question regarding alcohol consumption. In my past work as a GP Liaison Alcohol Counsellor within primary health, I placed strong emphasis on the role of nurses and health visitors in undertaking the initial screening that could identify an alcohol problem, and in training the members of primary healthcare teams in 'brief interventions', thereby enabling them to help a patient to acknowledge that they have a problem and to seek ways of changing their drinking pattern. If we are to extend alcohol screening and target brief intervention, the nurse in primary healthcare settings will have a key role.

What are brief interventions? Brief interventions are 'those practices that aim to identify an existing or potential alcohol problem and motivate an individual to do something about it'.[3] (p. 6) They are particularly suited for use in primary healthcare because of their being, as the name suggests, 'brief' interventions. In busy surgeries, there can be insufficient time to engage in protracted dialogue with patients with regard to their alcohol use. The need for a range of interventions that will offer maximum benefit from minimum time investment is crucially important. Of course, where more serious, enduring or complex alcohol problems are identified – alcohol dependence, traumatic psychological causes for alcohol use, co-morbidity with mental health or drug problems – then ideally the patient will be referred to specialist services that can offer more time within a multi-disciplinary framework. From my experience having a GP Liaison Alcohol or Substance Misuse professional within the surgery eases this process and enhances the likelihood of patients attending for further assessment and treatment.

The new-patient health check is an opportunity for questions to be asked about alcohol use, what has been termed 'universal screening'. Some surgeries may use a particular screening tool — for example, the Alcohol Use Disorders Identification Test (AUDIT). But it could be a locally produced set of questions. A surgery may have a policy of asking patients who attend at least once a year about their alcohol use, or may have certain 'trigger conditions' — alcohol related physical or mental health problems, a spouse with depression, children with behavioural problems — which will lead a member of the primary healthcare team to use a screening tool or to ask about alcohol use, the screening thereby being of a more 'targeted' nature. Whether a 'universal' or 'targeted' approach is followed, the goal remains that of identifying clients whose alcohol use is harmful or hazardous (above safe drinking limits).

From this it can be ascertained which clients have a level of drinking that may respond to brief interventions. It is important to target the intervention. Long-term chronic or dependent alcohol users are less likely to respond positively to brief interventions than is the person whose alcohol use has only been above safe drinking limits for a short period, or may have recently developed a problem that can be linked to their alcohol use: a physical injury, drink-driving, relationship problems, loss of a job. The person having recently turned to alcohol use to cope with a life-problem is likely to respond more favourably than the person drinking to cope with memories and psychological problems, for example associated with being the target of child sexual abuse. Those with a more ingrained alcohol habit including dependence (psychological and/or physical), and those for whom there is other complex symptomatology present, will need referral to specialist assessment and treatment services for longer term work.

There have been numerous randomised clinical trials of brief interventions over the past couple of decades, and in a variety of healthcare settings. Bien *et al.* considered 32 controlled studies which involved over 6000 patients, finding that 'there is encouraging evidence that the course of harmful alcohol use can be effectively altered by well-designed intervention strategies which are feasible within relatively brief-contact contexts such as primary healthcare setting and employee assistance programmes'.[4] More recent reviews have taken place, each also presenting positive evidence of brief interventions as being effective.[5-7]

Brief interventions (*see* Box 5.2) can range from five to ten minutes of screening, information and advice given to an excessive drinker; to two to three

---

Box 5.2   Six elements that have been shown to be effective in brief interventions, described using the 'FRAMES' model[10] (Bien *et al.* attributed to Miller and Sanchez)

F	feedback	assessment and evaluation of the problem
R	responsibility	emphasising that drinking is a choice
A	advice	explicit advice on changing drinking behaviour
M	menu	offering alternative goals and strategies
E	empathy	the role of the counsellor is important
S	self-efficacy	instilling optimism that the chosen goals can be achieved[4]

sessions of motivational interviewing or counselling.[8,9] They are usually opportunistic in the sense that a person has not specifically complained about an alcohol problem, but may be seeking help for reasons directly or indirectly associated with their alcohol use. The interventions involve a discussion on the patient's level of their pattern of alcohol use and how and why they might reduce consumption. The person's alcohol use is contrasted to 'safe-drinking benchmarks', average levels of drinking and the potential problems that can arise from heavy alcohol use. Goals may then be set for reducing consumption and the patient is encouraged to work towards this in a gradual and sustainable way. Sometimes leaflets and information sheets might be offered to encourage the patient further.

Stages of change

The motivational aspect of brief interventions should be emphasised and this is set against the 'cycle of change' model.[11] In this model, the process of change is defined in terms of different stages. These are:

- pre-contemplation
- contemplation
- preparation
- action
- maintenance
- relapse.

The stage the person is at with their alcohol use affects the nature and content of the responses made. The stages can be described in the following way.

Pre-contemplation
This stage represents the person, or pre-contemplator, who despite experiencing negative consequences of alcohol use does not regard themselves as having a problem and does not see any need to make changes to their alcohol use. The person is, quite simply, not thinking about change. Of course, they could be aware of a problem but are not prepared to admit it to anyone else for reasons perhaps of shame, or fear, the thought of the consequences of admitting to it and therefore accepting the need for treatment. The person in pre-contemplation needs to be given clear and unambiguous information, linking alcohol to any particular problems that have arisen. But do not push too much, this can tend to encourage resistance. In a sense the professional is sowing seeds in the mind of the patient. In a sense, the attempt is being made to unsettle the patient, help them to acknowledge that a problem, or potential problem, exists. This has to be done carefully and sensitively, leaving the patient aware that they can come back and discuss it further. Some patients will be made more anxious as they recognise that they have a problem but will refuse to admit it and simply go away and may even drink more. The patient needs to leave feeling that they can come back. The hope, however, will be that the pre-contemplator can be moved to begin to think about their alcohol use as being problematic, and want to address it.

Contemplation

The stage of contemplation is when the patient has begun to recognise that there is a problem with their alcohol use and needs to address it. They are, quite simply, now beginning to 'contemplate' change. At this point the patient is encouraged to look at their alcohol use, perhaps use a drinking diary to get a clearer idea of how much they drink, how much they spend, who they are with, what time they start, the contrast in their feelings before and after drinking. The drinking diary is a form of self-assessment for the client, but it can also be brought to the healthcare professional to discuss.

The patient will also be encouraged to weigh up the pros and cons of change. What are the advantages and disadvantages of change, and of not changing? These can be divided into short and longer term gains and losses. The gains are obviously motivating factors, but the losses need to be acknowledged as well as they provide potential lapse or relapse triggers and must be considered and catered for.

Another way of addressing this is through the use of a drinking life-line – the client is at a point of decision and two lines are drawn, like a fork in the road. One is the 'no change' line, the other is the 'change' line. Positive aspects of both choices are plotted above the two lines respectively, and negatives below them.[12] Again, it can offer a graphic image of the implications of the patient's choice to continue with their current level of drinking, or to reduce or even stop. And, of course, for some people the most telling aspect is that the life-line for change is more likely to be longer.

Preparation

As the person gains a clearer understanding of their alcohol use and of their need to make changes, then there comes a phase when they are preparing to put changes into operation. It is important to plan. The changes need to be clear and specific, measurable in the sense of an actual reduction in alcohol use, and monitored, for example with a drinking diary. Any risks to achieving what is being planned must be taken into account and planned for. Also, a clear timescale should be agreed. Where this seems impossible it could be that the patient actually does not yet want to change, has yet to really own the need and the planned process. They may still be contemplating and not yet ready for preparing.

Assume that the patient has the drinking pattern shown in Box 5.3.

Box 5.3   Example drinking pattern

- A beer at lunch times (2 units)
- A can of medium lager on the way home from work (2.5 units)
- A few beers in the pub in the evening (6 units)
- Followed by a 'nightcap' (2 units) at the end of the evening

This makes 12.5 units approximately in a day.

If the goal is to reduce to four units, but staged, the plan might be to stop the lunch time beer. Perhaps the person may do something else: eat in a café, go shopping, attempt a non-alcoholic alternative in the pub (perhaps the more difficult option for some). Or they may prefer to address the evening drinks and consider looking at an alternative activity some evenings to break up the habit of going to the pub. The patient might be encouraged to try to reduce or cut out the 'nightcap'. Alcohol disturbs sleep patterns. It does not induce quality sleep. Or the drink on the way home might be addressed; maybe they might try carrying a bottle of water or other drink (fizzy or fruit juice) if they are thirsty. The patient might also want to look at the the their routine on leaving work and see what alternatives there are.

Maybe there is a need for non-alcohol alternatives at home or when out; perhaps there is a need to reduce the actual strength of beer being consumed. There will be many ways to help the patient reduce their intake.

Whatever decisions are made, the following factors need to be in place.

- **S**pecific objectives that are clear are required.
- **M**easurable results should be obtained so that progress can be monitored.
- **A**greement – the client agrees and owns the plan and is committed to it.
- **R**ealism – it is vital that the client sees the plan as possible.
- **T**imescale must be clear for the client to put the plan into action.
- **Supportive** back-up should be planned and available.

What to do if a lapse or relapse occurs should also be discussed, so there is agreement as to what action the healthcare professional might initiate to contact the patient if they break contact.

Action
The action phase is, as the name suggests, the stage at which the patient acts on their plans for changing their alcohol intake. It will be a time when the patient will need support, perhaps a contact number for a local support line, or a short appointment to check-in and receive encouragement. It is often said in the world of alcohol treatment that it is not change that is difficult, it is sustaining change. But so long as the possible relapse triggers have been identified and the patient truly and genuinely owns their action plan, there is every reason to hope that they will be able to make progress in the planned changes.

Maintenance
How long does it take someone to maintain a change to their drinking before it can be deemed sustainable? In the example above, the person may, over a few weeks, have gradually reduced their intake and achieved the target of approximately four units a day. They do not want to change further, but now they must sustain this and ensure that it does not creep back up. What will be required for them to maintain their change? They are now drinking only some evenings in the pub, and on the evenings that they don't, they have a couple of cans at home.

If they drink at some other time of the day they will need to be willing to adjust to maintain their four-unit maximum. They will need to continue the changes of routine that they have established at lunch time and in travelling home from work. They will need to sustain changes, perhaps, in their social life, and of having a different routine last thing at night. How will they cope with celebrations when they may drink more? Will they seek a reduced alcohol day the next day or for more days to keep the weekly total down? And if it was to creep up, at what point might they seek help and support once more, and perhaps a reassessment of the situation and of possible treatment needs to help them further if it turns out that they simply cannot sustain the lower alcohol intake?

The length of time that people can spend in maintenance can vary. Often the patient will know, although there is a risk that people can seek to test themselves, particularly when someone has decided to aim for abstinence but then thinks that just the odd drink will be 'OK'. For some people it can be OK, but for others, it can lead to a return to the previous pattern, or worse.

Relapse

It may seem strange that relapse appears in a cycle of change, however it has its place. In fact, it can be considered in terms of lapse or relapse. Lapse is more of a 'blip'; a relapse is a return to the original pattern. In helping someone at this stage it can be about encouraging them in such a way as to stop a lapse becoming a relapse. Perhaps something unplanned happened. Perhaps the person had been drinking more than they have said, and are actually experiencing a withdrawal reaction that makes it difficult if not impossible (and dangerous) for them to sustain their planned reduction. Perhaps the plan wasn't wholly owned by the patient – it was more something that the well-meaning health professional organised them into doing, but which the patient was not really ready for.

The patient at this stage can be very low in mood, feeling hopeless and helpless. They may break contact. At the preparation stage, what to do if a lapse or relapse occurs needs to be planned for. Will the patient simply be left to make contact? Better that there is an agreement for the healthcare professional to instigate contact, and in as sensitive a way as possible given the way that the patient may be feeling.

Sustaining change

Some people will need more than one attempt before their change is sustained. Others may exit from maintenance on the first attempt to change their drinking pattern. Others will break contact in relapse and may not present again for a while. Yet the idea of brief interventions offered within the framework of the cycle of change, and with an underlying agenda of seeking to encourage motivation in the patient to change, has been demonstrated to be effective. The nurse working in primary care will have a key role in facilitating the change.

Summary

Aspects of the *Alcohol Harm Reduction Strategy for England* have been outlined, with reference to healthcare. There is a recognised need for a more concerted and co-ordinated approach to changing the culture of drinking in England, to provide screening and assessment in a variety of health, social care, criminal justice and other settings, to ensure that a range of evidence based treatment responses is available with professionals suitably trained – including brief interventions in primary healthcare settings.

It is unfortunate that the Government believes there is a need to collect further evidence as to the effectiveness of brief interventions, and that it is not releasing further funding to enable services to expand in order to cater for the demand for alcohol treatment (a demand that is likely to grow given the increasing consumption of alcohol, particularly amongst young people), and to end the problems associated with short-term funding that makes long-term planning so difficult.

The existence of the *Alcohol Harm Reduction Strategy for England* must be regarded as a step forward. We have a framework to work within. It will involve collaboration from all sections of society and encouragement of greater responsibility for the individual when it comes to alcohol use. It will require the drinks industry to consider the effects of its products and the manner of its marketing. It will require integrated pathways of care established between services – both alcohol specialist and non-specialist – and with clear referral links from other bodies including education, criminal justice and social services.

Alcohol affects people of all ages. You do not have to be a problem drinker to experience problematic effects of alcohol use. You could be the person bumping into the wrong person leaving a pub at 11.00 pm who pulls a knife in a moment of drunken belligerence. Or you could be the two-year-old whose head hits the corner of the glass table-top after being dropped by a parent who loses their balance after a second bottle of wine at home, or the unborn child damaged by a mother's drinking during pregnancy. English social life has, to some degree, become dependent on alcohol. We must hope that the *Alcohol Harm Reduction Strategy for England* proves to be a watershed, demonstrating an admittance that there is a problem, that not only must change be contemplated, but actually prepared for in the hope that a sustainable change to the English drinking culture in the decades ahead can be maintained.

References

1   Strategy Unit (2004) *Alcohol Harm Reduction Strategy for England.* Cabinet Office, London.
2   Alcohol Concern (2004) *Response to the National Alcohol Harm Reduction Strategy.* Alcohol Concern, London.
3   Babor TF and Higgins-Biddle JL (2001) *Brief Intervention for Hazardous and Harmful Drinking: a manual for use in primary care.* WHO, Geneva.
4   Bien TH, Miller WR and Tonigan JS (1993) Brief interventions for alcohol problems: a review. *Addiction.* **88**: 315–36.
5   Kahan M, Wilson L and Becker L (1995) Effectiveness of physician-based interventions with problem drinkers: a review. *Canadian Medical Association Journal.* **152**: 851–9.
6   Wilk AI, Jensen MN and Havighurst TC (1997) Meta-analysis of randomized control trials addressing brief interventions in heavy alcohol drinkers. *Archives of Internal Medicine.* **12**: 274–83.
7   Poikolainen K (1999) Effectiveness of brief interventions to reduce alcohol intake in primary health care populations: a meta-analysis. *Preventative Medicine.* **28**: 503–9.

8   Miller WR and Rollnick S (1991) *Motivational Interviewing: preparing people to change addictive behaviour.* Guilford Press, New York.

9   Alcohol Concern (2001) *Factsheet 15: Brief Interventions.* Alcohol Concern, London.

10 Miller WR and Sanchez VC (1993) Motivating young adults for treatment and lifestyle change. In: G Howard (ed.) *Issues in Alcohol Use and Misuse in Young Adults.* University of Notre Dame Press, Notre Dame, IN.

11 Prochaska JO and DiClemente CC (1986) Towards a comprehensive model of change. In: WR Miller and N Heather (eds) *Treating Addictive Behaviours: processes of change.* Plenum, New York.

12 Bryant-Jefferies R (2001) *Counselling the Person Beyond the Alcohol Problem.* Jessica Kingsley, London.

CHAPTER 6

The role of the midwife working with a pregnant drug user

Catherine Barnard Siney

Introduction

The role of the midwife has evolved in recent years with more emphasis on a public health role.[1] Midwives can feel that they need to know everything about everything. This is not actually so but it is reasonable to expect that midwives should have a working knowledge of the effects of drugs that are illicit and those that can be prescribed and are misused, as well as other common public health issues, including teenage pregnancy, alcohol abuse, smoking and obesity. They should have an understanding of the common risks associated with drug and/or alcohol dependency and what they should be able to offer by way of support.[2] Accurate record-keeping is essential so that audit can be used to identify any additional needs as well as ensuring that the women and their families receive good quality appropriate care and advice.

Key points

- You do not need to be a 'specialist' to discuss the potential risks of substance misuse and you can use a leaflet to help you describe what this means clinically.
- You must have details of local support/treatment agencies for drug addiction to hand and if the woman wishes, you should make the call for her to the appropriate service.
- It is important to remember that patterns of substance misuse vary around the country so management of the womens' problems and their babies will also vary. Consensus on management can be very difficult to achieve even within one maternity unit, therefore management plans for both women and babies should be agreed, consistently carried out and audited at least annually.

This chapter covers the following key areas.

- Identification of women with drug/alcohol dependency issues.
- Problems of non-identification.
- Screening for drug misuse.
- Risks/complications of dependency relating to pregnancy.

- Inter-agency working, confidentiality and child protection.
- Antenatal care.
- Labour and delivery care.
- Postnatal care for mother and baby and breastfeeding.

Identification

Women who are drug and/or alcohol dependent may not be obviously so, although some women may fulfil the stereotypes that we see in the media. Women who do not identify themselves and ask for advice, help or support are not necessarily uncaring about the pregnancy. There are many reasons for the women not to disclose this information, many relating to the attitudes of professionals or at least the perceived attitudes of professionals – with particular concern about social services – or fear of the expectations that the professionals will have about the effect of pregnancy on their dependency.

Some women may not know about the risks and some may feel very guilty and think that the risks are too horrible to think about so do not wish to discuss them. Other women may fear that they will be judged as bad parents and automatically referred to social services. Some may have had experience of children being removed by social services because of their drug taking. The attitude of social services has changed over time, however many professionals from both health and social care still feel that there should be a child protection case conference whenever any drug use is mentioned (*see* Chapter 7).[3]

It is important for midwives to be non-judgemental. The amount of drugs taken and the frequency of drug use will vary greatly. Many women use drugs occasionally, and only a small number will become dependent and it is important that women feel able to tell midwives about any substance they are using so that they can be given accurate advice. Pregnancy and birth should be as positive an experience for the women as possible. This is as important as achieving a healthy mother and a healthy baby at the end of the pregnancy.

Problems of non-identification

The following list shows the problems of non-identification.

- Inadequate support for this vulnerable group of women.
- Inability to inform the woman of the risks she may be running with both her health and that of her baby.
- No chance for the woman to make changes to her lifestyle.
- No chance for assessment of parenting needs in the light of her dependency.
- No chance to gather information to assess the need for referral to social services if there is a child or children in need of protection.

Screening for substance misuse

All women should be asked about the use of substances as part of antenatal history taking. Consistency of recording is important, along with the number of tobacco cigarettes smoked daily, alcohol should be recorded as units weekly taking into

Box 6.1   **Example question on alcohol consumption in antenatal history taking**

Question: How many units of alcohol do you drink a week?

Answer: (1–10)   (11+)
(*Delete as appropriate*)

Advice: (dependent on answer)
'It is preferable not to drink alcohol whilst pregnant (or indeed if planning pregnancy) but:

- 1–10 units   should not be drunk all at one time
- 11+   this level may be OK when not pregnant but may be linked to foetal alcohol syndrome (FAS)/foetal alcohol effects (FAE)
- Dependency   is linked to FAS.'

If a woman has been referred with a history of dependency then it is important to record information about past or current management of the dependence.

account the strength of various drinks. There is good evidence to show that women respond accurately to specific questions and this enables women who may have a problem to be identified even if they do not think they have one (*see* Chapter 4).[4] A sample question for use during antenatal history taking is shown in Box 6.1 together with some advice.[5] The answers to questions about smoking and alcohol should be followed up each time a woman is seen for antenatal care since circumstances can change during the course of a pregnancy.

The *Confidential Enquiry into Maternal Deaths* (2000) flagged the large proportion of women who had had a drug problem as well as reminding us of the link between socio-economic deprivation and poorer outcomes in pregnancy.[6] It is essential therefore that every woman is asked about drug use at her booking appointment. The question 'Have you ever taken any unprescribed drugs?' is simple to ask and allows the woman to know that this is a routine question and she can feel safe to admit that she is now taking or has taken unprescribed drugs. Box 6.2 shows a flowchart of questions if the woman answers positively. It is important to acknowledge that the questions are not being asked for moral or legal reasons but for health reasons.

A past history of non-injecting drug taking may not be clinically important in itself but may indicate that the woman might need additional support at times of stress or crisis.

Obviously a current history of regular drug use, whether dependent or not may need to be dealt with by the offer of professional drug counselling.

A past or current history of injecting drug use is of clinical significance since it opens the women to the risk of testing positive for a bloodborne virus and the risk of passing this to their baby (*see* Box 6.3 and Chapter 4).

Box 6.2   Antenatal history questions for all women

Question: Have you ever taken any unprescibed drugs?

Answer: Yes   No
(*Delete as appropriate*)

If **No** ⟶ No further questions/action.
If **Yes** ⟶

Question: If you are currently taking them or have recently stopped would you like some help?

Answer: Yes   No

If **No** ⟶ **Advice**: 'I think it's important for you to understand the risks to you and your baby. Here is a leaflet with contact numbers for the specialist midwife [*if there is one*]/local drug/counselling agency. It also has information about the risks and what to expect from the maternity service.'
If **Yes** ⟶ Referral to drug/counselling agency and specialist midwife [*if there is one*].
⟶ give leaflet about what the woman should expect from the maternity service and read it with her.

Question: Did you ever inject?

Answer: Yes   No

If **No** ⟶ No further action
If **Yes** ⟶ It is important to discuss BBVs (bloodborne viruses) and the risks of vertical transmission (*see* Box 6.4).

Question: What drugs are you taking now (or if stopped only recently – when stopped)?

Answer:			
Opiates (e.g. heroin, 'DF118')		Yes	No
Cocaine (including 'crack')		Yes	No
Benzodiazepines (e.g. temazepam, diazepam)		Yes	No
Amphetamines (including ecstasy)		Yes	No
Cannabis (in any form)		Yes	No
Anything else – please state			

Question: Have you, or are you, receiving help from an agency – if so what is its name?

Box 6.4 shows a flowchart of antenatal history questions for women who are referred as drug dependent. These should be asked in addition to the questions about injecting and what drugs are being used currently. A checklist at the inside front cover of the hospital records allows everyone to see that communication

Box 6.3   Vertical transmission risk of bloodborne viruses

HIV (human immunodeficiency virus):[17]
- Approximately 25% chance of vertical transmission if the woman is asymptomatic and has no treatment.
- Risk is reduced to < 5% if the woman is treated with current drug therapy.
- May be increased if the woman is symptomatic or if she breastfeeds.
- Preferable mode of delivery is caesarian section.

HBV (hepatitis B):[18]
- 70–90% dependent on whether the woman is of low or high infectivity.
- The infant will require the post-exposure schedule for vaccination, i.e. birth, one month, two months and a booster and blood test at 12 months.
- The infant may require HBV specific immunoglobulin (as well as vaccination) if the woman is of high infectivity.

HCV (hepatitis C):[19]
- 5+% dependent on co-infection with HIV.
- The infant will require blood testing to exclude infection usually at six, 12 and 18 months.

Box 6.4   Antenatal history – additional questions for women referred as drug dependent

Question: Who are you receiving treatment/counselling from?

Answer: Drug dependency unit/GP/community drug team/other e.g. DTTO (drug treatment and testing order)
(*Delete as appropriate and give telephone number and keyworker name*)

Question: What medication are you on (if any)?

_____

Question: What is the plan for prescribing in pregnancy?

_____

Qustion: Is your health visitor (HV) aware of your pregnancy or dependency or both?

_____

(If this is a first baby the HV should be informed as soon as possible. If this is not a first baby the HV should have been informed by the prescriber – you should check.)

Continued

> **Question**:   Have you now or have you ever had social service involvement?
>
> **Question**:   If current involvement is she/he aware of this pregnancy?
>
> It is important that women who misuse drugs/alcohol know that they are not viewed automatically as a 'bad parent' and referred to social services.[3,12] They should be given information about the maternity services, and also what the local policy is for pre-birth risk assessment. (If you do not know what the local policy is you should contact your named midwife/nurse for child protection.)

between professionals has been achieved – it also allows the management to be audited. This in turn allows statistics to be made into an annual report to be shared with all interested agencies.

Risks/complications of dependency

It is important to remember that women with a dependency may not be in the best of general health (*see* Chapters 4 and 5). This and a poor diet affect the pregnancy in common with any chronic health problem. Risks associated with drug misuse such as overdose and withdrawal; an increased rate of dental caries; respiratory problems; subcutaneous, deep, mycotic and septicaemic infections; and trauma-induced injury from injecting drug use continue.[7]

Specific drug effects

The effects of a specific drug on a pregnant woman and her foetus are considered.

Opiates
Amenorrhoea is common among opiate dependent women therefore making the dating of pregnancy difficult. The late booking that this can cause makes dating by ultrasound inaccurate. There is an increased risk of antepartum haemorrhage due both to placental abruption and placenta praevia. Gestational hypertension and breech presentation are also reportedly increased. It is unclear whether this is specific to opiates or a reflection of general poor health and socio-economic circumstances. The most consistently reported findings are an increased incidence of pre-term deliveries and small-for-gestational-age babies. Opiates do not appear to increase the risk of congenital abnormalities but babies will experience symptoms of withdrawal to a lesser or greater degree and some may require pharmaceutical management as well as comfort measures and regular as opposed to demand feeding. Generally babies are small-for-gestational-age and require frequent regular feeding.[8]

Cocaine
Cocaine in any form is a vasoconstrictor and is associated with maternal hypertension, spontaneous abortion and placental abruption. Intrauterine growth retardation (IUGR) is the most consistent finding in all studies, it is interesting to note that, unlike the IUGR caused by opiates, brain growth can be impaired as well.[8,9]

Benzodiazepines

The effects of benzodiazepines on pregnancy are uncertain but the use of diazepam in early pregnancy has been associated with an increased incidence of cleft palate, and doses of more than 30 mg per day may result in withdrawal symptoms in the baby.[8,10]

Amphetamines

There is no good evidence of any link between amphetamine use and congenital abnormalities, although their use in pregnancy is not uncommon.[11]

Alcohol

Chronic alcohol abuse can cause foetal alcohol syndrome (FAS). This diagnosis requires signs in three categories: foetal growth retardation, central nervous system involvement (neurological abnormalities, developmental delay, intellectual impairment, etc.) and facial deformity. A small proportion of heavy drinkers give birth to babies with FAS, a lesser syndrome is known as foetal alcohol effects (FAE).[11]

Research is consistent in finding no evidence of foetal harm in pregnant women who drink fewer than ten units per week providing that the drink is taken over several days and not all at once. Frequent drinkers are defined as women who drink more than ten units per week but who are not alcohol dependent. These women may be at risk of having a baby with FAE. Foetal alcohol syndrome occurs in babies born to women who are dependent on alcohol. They are likely to consume at least six units of alcohol every day. Moderate to heavy alcohol intake during pregnancy is associated with an increased risk of spontaneous abortion and stillbirths.[12]

It is important to remember that there may be multiple effects on the health of a pregnant woman due to poor socio-economic circumstances and tobacco smoking in addition to the substance misuse. Of course, all the usual risks and complications of pregnancy also apply.

Inter-agency working, confidentiality and child protection

Midwives are used to working with other healthcare providers when planning care for women with complex physical needs but may not feel quite so confident when working with non-health agencies, e.g. prison services, probation services or social services.

If a woman is already known to be drug/alcohol dependent and attending a treatment programme, then the GP will probably have detailed key contacts in their referral letter to the consultant at the hospital, or the agency may well have sent information directly if they know the woman is pregnant, either way it is essential for all or anyone involved in treating the woman to be in regular communication. Drug prescribers should always notify the hospital of any prescription changes to ensure continuity for hospital admissions and any changes in the woman's dependency should always be communicated. Box 6.5 shows a communication flowchart.

It is as well to remember that for long-term drug/alcohol dependent women, pregnancy may not make as huge an impact on lifestyle as you would hope or

---

Box 6.5   Communication flowchart for maternity service

Woman: _____

(known or identified)

Booking appointment:	Letter to GP (copy to HV and to prescriber)
Anomaly scan:	Letter to GP (copy to HV and to prescriber)
Growth scan (28/40) and ANC appointment:	Letter to GP (copy to HV and to prescriber)
Growth scan (34/40) and ANC appointment:	Letter to GP confirming any drug dosage as related by patient and any plans made by social services about parenting issues (copy to HV and to prescriber)
Admission for delivery:	Telephone call to prescriber
Postnatal discharge:	Verbal information to HV and prescribers Letter to GP copied to HV and prescribers

---

think. In my experience women may modify their behaviours, but it is unlikely to cure them of their dependency. For professionals and indeed the women themselves to have that expectation may lead to a lot of disappointment and feelings of failure which are not useful. What should be expected is a modification of lifestyle indicated by a reduction in illicit drug use and/or a reduction in prescribed drugs demonstrating some understanding of the realities and responsibilities of parenting.

The prescribing or treatment agency will be assessing the effects of the dependency on potential parenting ability and this should be communicated to other health carers. This does not mean that midwives have no responsibilities around assessment of parenting ability. Any drug/alcohol dependent woman who turned up at an antenatal appointment and appeared unsteady or who was very sleepy or slurred their speech would need to be discussed very quickly with social services. Similarly a woman who was booked for antenatal care and then stopped attending would need urgent referral also provided, of course, she has not had a miscarriage or termination of pregnancy.

When a woman is pregnant the situation should be discussed with the health visitor (HV) so that she/he is able to undertake a pre-birth risk assessment. The HV may not know that the woman is misusing drugs or alcohol although it would be good practice for any provider of treatment programmes to notify the HV if a client has care of children (even if they are not their own).

If a midwife is unsure about child protection issues then she should speak to her named midwife who will be able to advise. The named midwife (or alternatively the named nurse for child protection) is a senior midwife/nurse who has undertaken training in child protection and she will be able to support her if she needs to make a referral to social services without the permission of the woman.

Confidentiality policies are always overridden if a child is in need of protection, but it should be remembered that being a drug dependent parent or potential parent does not automatically make someone a bad parent and that each case needs to be assessed individually (*see* Chapter 7).[3]

Antenatal care
Frequency/venues

Antenatal care for this group of women should occur whenever possible! This acknowledges that a number of drug/alcohol dependent women are likely to be unreliable in their attendance at antenatal appointments. Monthly antenatal care at any venue by anyone qualified is a simple system as listed.[13]

- Prescribing clinic, by a midwife.
- GP surgery, by a GP or midwife.
- 'Drop-in' centres/needle and syringe exchanges, by a midwife.
- Hospital clinic, by an obstetrician. (Attendance at ultrasound departments also counts.)

It is important to keep good records ensuring that all agencies involved with care are kept up to date. Great care must be taken that hand-held records do not contain anything the woman does not want. Family members who are not aware of the situation may look at the records or they may be lost. Confidential information should be retained in the hospital records with some sort of agreed symbol on the hand-held records that would indicate that there is relevant information in the hospital record. Most units will have a way of indicating confidential information, e.g. terminations of pregnancy or mental health problems or a child being adopted, and substance misuse should be included as confidential information.

Similarly, special antenatal clinics may appear to the women to identify them as deviating from 'normal' pregnant women. Integrating them into a 'high risk' clinic would solve that issue.

Screening

All the routine blood tests are appropriate. However, it is important to remember that women who may have injected or had a partner who has injected would be considered in a high risk category for bloodborne viruses (BBVs). If you do not feel that you have sufficient expertise to discuss the prospect of a positive test then there should be easy access to counselling for BBVs usually at the GUM (genitourinary medicine) department unless there is a specialist midwife/nurse available. Women who have had a long-term dependency problem and have accessed specialist services will usually have had BBVs discussed at length and will have already been offered testing.

Information about BBVs test results will be shared by other health services as should any antenatal blood test results (*see* Chapter 4).

Constipation

Constipation is a cause for concern in opiate dependent women because the abdominal pain associated with it may lead the woman to believe she is miscarrying (if in early pregnancy) or in early labour. Discussion about diet and fluids may be useful but bowel habits should be enquired about regularly throughout pregnancy and aperients may be required.

Prescribing in pregnancy

An overall reduction in prescribed, illicit and legal (i.e. tobacco) drugs is the aim in pregnancy, whilst maintaining the woman's ability to parent. Therefore it is important to have realistic expectations of what is achievable for the woman. She should be reassured that whatever medication she is prescribed will be continued during any admission to hospital. There should be clear communication about continued use of any drugs on top of prescribed medication by the pregnant woman (*see* Chapter 2 for information about management of dependency).

It is important to note that approximately 10% of all pregnancies end in the first trimester so that this is incorporated into plans for drug detoxification. Also towards the end of pregnancy with the large increase in blood volume, plans for management may need to be amended. The aim for prescribing in pregnancy is stability leading to some reduction in use and dependency.

Onset of labour/complications in pregnancy

It is essential that pregnant women are told that if they have stomach pains they should have them checked by a healthcare professional. Withdrawal symptoms from opiates include stomach cramps so it is important that women do not put themselves or their babies at risk by assuming that any stomach cramps are from withdrawals. Similarly it should be emphasised that any loss from the vagina should be investigated.

Women who are injecting drug users should be advised to see their drug service for advice in order to ensure that they do not inject into breast veins if they are unable to access their groin injection sites.

Labour and delivery

Opiate levels need to be maintained so that routine analgesia will work and the risk of an unnecessary caesarian section or foetal blood sampling is reduced. The paediatricians should be notified of the labour, though it may not be necessary to attend the birth. Naloxone should be used with care in the knowledge that its use may precipitate rapid withdrawal symptoms in the newborn.[14]

Postnatal care

Following delivery, babies should remain with their mothers unless there is a medical reason for admission to a special care baby unit, or the child is being removed from the care of the mother by court order.

Babies who have symptoms of withdrawal following delivery require a lot of one-to-one care and the only person available to do this is the mother. Therefore mothers and babies should be on a postnatal ward together, where monitoring and any treatment should take place. Even if a baby does not require treatment she/he will require non-subjective monitoring and a lot of cuddling and feeding. Care should be taken to exclude other reasons for any symptoms, e.g. hypoglycaemia, before treatment is commenced.[14]

If treatment is 'comfort and not sedation' then this enables the mother to continue to be the main carer for her child. The pharmaceutical treatment of babies who need it appears to remain inconsistent across maternity units. It would be useful if units audited their plans of management and shared them at least regionally. This would allow larger units to share their findings with smaller units.

Babies not being treated should be discharged home as early as possible even if they still exhibit symptoms. If treatment is commenced it should be completed before discharge. It should be emphasised to the woman and her family that any problems following discharge should be discussed with the midwife, GP or HV as usual.

Information about treatment or vaccination should be communicated to the GP and HV. Depending on maternal HBV (hepatitis B virus) status the baby may require HBV specific immunoglobulin as well as the post-exposure schedule of HBV vaccinations, i.e. birth, one month, two months and a booster and blood test at 12 months. The woman should have been referred to a hepatologist for follow-up. If the woman is HCV (hepatitis C virus) positive both she and the baby will require follow-up. If the woman is HIV (human immunodeficiency virus) positive, she will have been offered treatment during pregnancy. If she accepts it, this will have continued during delivery and the baby will be followed-up with blood testing in the community (*see* Chapter 4).

Breastfeeding

Opiates/opioids
The available evidence suggests that methadone (a heroin substitute), morphine and diamorphine (pharmaceutical grade heroin) are unlikely to cause harm to the baby unless the mother is taking exceptionally large doses, nevertheless there is a risk of accumulation with prolonged exposure because they are metabolised very slowly by the infant. Heroin is adulterated with other substances and therefore could pose a risk to the baby.[15]

Cocaine
Women should not breastfeed since the drug can pass into breastmilk and may be concentrated there, causing adverse effects including irritability and hypertension.[15]

Benzodiazepines
There are reports of sedation in babies who have also been exposed antenatally.[10]

Amphetamines
There is very limited data available. It is possible that regular high-dose amphetamine might impair milk production. It is therefore advisable, because of lack of data, that regular amphetamine users should not breastfeed.

Alcohol

The effects of alcohol on the infant are not clear but women should restrict their intake whilst breastfeeding. Regular high intake of alcohol may suppress milk supply, however, even small amounts of alcohol may reduce the amount of milk consumed by an infant by a quarter.[12]

It is important when giving advice about breastfeeding and drugs and alcohol that women may be taking more than one drug.

Women who are HIV positive are advised against breastfeeding but women who are HBV positive are advised that breastfeeding is not thought to be important in mother–baby transmission.[16] Women who are HCV positive should not be discouraged from breastfeeding, but advice may be required from a virologist if there is viraemia. Mother to baby transmission of HCV is usually low.

Summary

Caring for pregnant women who are drug/alcohol dependent can appear daunting but we, as midwives, are used to managing women with complex needs in partnership with other agencies. A 'user friendly' service enables the women to have some control over their situation – about where to have antenatal care and also about what to do about their drug use. It also means that they will have information about what to expect during their pregnancy and postnatally.

The following is a list of points to remember:

* communication
  – between professionals
  – between professionals/pregnant women
* honesty
  – realistic expectations for both women and professionals
  – the truth about risks of drugs and childcare concerns
* respect
  – for the women and their choices (whether we approve or not)
  – for the opinions of all those who work with these vulnerable women.

References

1 Department of Health (1993) *Expert Maternity Group: changing childbirth*. HMSO, London.
2 English National Board (2001) *Midwives in Action: a resource*. English National Board (ENB), Victory House, London. (Now Nurses and Midwives Board.)
3 SCODA (1997) *Drug-Using Parents: policy guidelines for inter-agency working*. Local Government Drug Forum.
4 Clarke KA, Dawson S and Martin SL (1999) The effect of implementing a more comprehensive screening for substance use among pregnant women in North Carolina. *Maternal and Child Health Journal*. **3**(3): 161–6. Abstracted in: *MIDIRS Midwifery Digest* (2000) **10**: 3.
5 Department of Health (1995) *Sensible Drinking. The Report of an Interdepartmental Working Group*. HMSO, London.

6   Department of Health (2000) *Confidential Enquiry into Maternal Deaths.* HMSO, London.

7   Morrison CL (1999) The medical problems of illicit drug use in pregnancy and harm minimisation. In: C Siney (ed.) *Pregnancy and Drug Misuse.* Books for Midwives Press, pp. 43–53.

8   Sparey C and Walkinshaw S (1999) Obstetric problems for drug users. In: C Siney (ed.) *Pregnancy and Drug Misuse.* Books for Midwives Press, pp. 55–68.

9   The Northern Neonatal Network (2000) *Neonatal Formulary 3.* BMJ Books, London, p. 252.

10   The Northern Neonatal Network (2000) *Neonatal Formulary 3.* BMJ Books, London, p. 92.

11   Mounteney J (1999) *Drugs, Pregnancy and Childcare.* Institute for the Study of Drug Dependence, London, pp. 12–32.

12   Wills S (2000) Social drugs. In: A Lee, S Inch and D Finnigan (eds) *Therapeutics in Pregnancy and Lactation.* Radcliffe Medical Press, Oxford, pp. 215–18.

13   Siney C, Kidd M, Walkinshaw S *et al.* (1995) Opiate dependency and pregnancy. *British Journal of Midwifery.* **3**(2): 69–73.

14   Shaw B (1999) Maternal drug use: consequences for the child. In: C Siney (ed.) *Pregnancy and Drug Misuse.* Books for Midwives Press, pp. 69–79.

15   Wills S (2000) Street drugs. In: A Lee, S Inch and D Finnigan (eds) *Therapeutics in Pregnancy and Lactation.* Radcliffe Medical Press, Oxford, pp. 227–46.

16   Carey P (1999) Hepatitis B, pregnancy and the drug user and HIV. In: C Siney (ed.) *Pregnancy and Drug Misuse.* Books for Midwives Press, pp. 81–106.

17   British HIV Association (2001) *Guidelines for the Management of HIV Infection in Pregnant Women and the Prevention of Mother to Child Transmission.* Blackwell Science, Oxford.

18   Ballard AL and Boxall EH (1999) Assessing the infectivity of hepatitis B carriers. *Comm Dis Public Health.* **2**: 78–83.

19   Hadžić N (2001) Hepatitis C in pregnancy. *Archives of Diseases in Childhood (Fetal Neonatal Edition).* **84**: F201–4.

CHAPTER 7

The role of the health visitor in relation to child protection and substance misuse

Claire Chambers, Marguerite Williams and *Bernie Halford*

Introduction

Many children have suffered severe abuse at the hands of their parents and problematic drug use is often a contributory factor. Some of this abuse has tragically resulted in the death of a child. In a series of 13 Serious Case Reviews, conducted as a result of a child's death, four children experienced substance misuse as a major contributory factor.[1] This chapter discusses the role of the health visitor (HV) in assessing and attempting to address the needs of parents and their children when substance misuse is part of their lives. The principles of health visiting will be used as a framework for the chapter, which will explore how HVs need to use a multi-agency approach in order to address these needs.[2] Case studies will be used to discuss the various aspects of the care of a family where problem drug use is involved, and reflective points will be made throughout to focus the reader's thoughts on practice issues.

Hidden Harm: responding to the needs of children of problem drug users highlights the concerning statistics in relation to parental problem drug use.[3] The parents of 2–3% of all children under the age of 16 years in England and Wales, and 4–6% of all children in Scotland are classed as problem drug users.[3] (p. 20) The document states that 'there was clear evidence that the more severe the parents' drug problems, the more likely they are to be separated from their children'.[3] (p. 90) The report makes the point that 'if 2–3% of children in England and Wales are affected but parental problem drug use is a major contributory factor in 20% or more of the cases on the child protection register, that in itself is an indication of the potential for serious harm'.[3] (p. 90) Box 7.1 lists the six key messages from the report.[3]

The immense effect of parental problem drug use on children is clearly expressed in the report which states that this has the 'potential to disturb every aspect of a child's development from conception onwards'.[3] (p. 90) Harbin and Murphy highlight various factors associated with this higher risk to children as shown in Box 7.2.

Box 7.1 Six key messages from *Hidden Harm*[3]

- There are between 250 000 and 350 000 children of problem drug users in the UK — about one for every problem drug user.
- Parental problem drug use can and does cause serious harm to children at every age from conception to adulthood.
- Reducing the harm to children from parental problem drug use should become a main objective of policy and practice.
- Effective treatment of the parent can have major benefits for the child.
- By working together, services can take many practical steps to protect and improve the health and wellbeing of affected children.
- The number of affected children is only likely to decrease when the number of problem drug users decreases.

Box 7.2 Factors associated with higher risk to children[4]

- Addicted parent being the mother.
- Longer period of drug use.
- Continuing substance misuse.
- Continuing substance misuse in pregnancy.
- Use of other drugs in addition to methadone.
- Drug taking affecting lifestyle.
- Greater degree of poverty.
- Presence of domestic violence.
- Lack of social support.
- Lower parental education and learning difficulties.
- Very young mothers (aged under 18) and mothers aged over 30.
- Infant withdrawal symptoms.
- Previous child abuse.
- Previous child in care.
- Poor parenting skills, for example in child discipline and knowledge of child development.

Definitions of child abuse

Children whose parent/s are problem drug users can be at risk of any form of child abuse; however physical abuse, emotional abuse, sexual abuse and neglect can be particular risks for these children (Box 7.3).

Neglect is very closely linked with substance misuse and a study carried out by Savage showed that 75% of mothers in the sample seriously misused alcohol and as a result interaction with their children was largely absent.[6] There was a severe lack of supervision and guidance, and physical and emotional neglect was a fundamental part of their childrens' lives. Parents in this situation suffer from low

---

Box 7.3   *Working Together to Safeguard Children*: definition of child abuse[5] (pp. 5–6)

Physical abuse: May involve hitting, shaking, throwing, poisoning, burning or scalding, drowning, suffocating or otherwise causing physical harm to a child. Physical harm may also be caused when a parent or carer feigns the symptoms of, or deliberately causes ill health to a child whom they are looking after. This situation is commonly described using terms such as factitious illness by proxy or Münchausen syndrome by proxy.

Emotional abuse: Is the persistent emotional ill-treatment of a child such as to cause severe and persistent adverse effects on the child's emotional development. It may involve conveying to children that they are worthless or unloved, inadequate, or valued only insofar as they meet the needs of another person. It may feature age or developmentally inappropriate expectations being imposed on children. It may involve causing children frequently to feel frightened or in danger, or the exploitation or corruption of children. Some level of emotional abuse is involved in all types of ill-treatment of a child, though it may occur alone.

Sexual abuse: Involves forcing or enticing a child or young person to take part in sexual activities, whether or not the child is aware of what is happening. The activities may involve physical contact, including penetrative (e.g. rape or buggery) or non-penetrative acts. They may include non-contact activities, such as involving children in looking at, or in the production of, pornographic material or watching sexual activities, or encouraging children to behave in sexually inappropriate ways.

Neglect: Is the persistent failure to meet a child's basic physical and/or psychological needs, likely to result in the serious impairment of the child's health or development. It may involve a parent or carer failing to provide adequate food, shelter and clothing; failing to protect a child from physical harm or danger; or failure to ensure access to appropriate medical care or treatment. It may also include neglect of, or unresponsiveness to, a child's basic emotional needs.

---

self-esteem and a poor internal locus of control and are often unable to motivate themselves to cope with their lives and their childrens' needs, or provide the quality of care that promotes adequate development and wellbeing.

Browne *et al.* discuss the links between mental health problems, domestic violence, child abuse and substance misuse.[7] They state that while drug and alcohol misuse appear to exacerbate pre-existing factors such as domestic violence and emotional or mental health problems, and can co-exist together, the substance misuse can also be used as an excuse for their violent behaviour. Therefore all these factors have to be perceived as risk factors in relation to the safety of children.

Legislative framework in relation to child protection

It is important to ensure that the children of problem drug users are perceived as children at risk of significant harm, and that they receive early identification and multi-agency support to prevent end-stage crisis intervention which is often the case in the current financial climate. However, it is also important that substance misuse is not perceived as an automatic indicator of significant harm.

The Children Act 1989 provides a framework for the care and protection of children and outlines a number of general principles which need to be borne in mind when considering the legal framework.[8]

Box 7.4   General principles when applying a legal framework to child protection situations

- The welfare of the child is paramount.[s1 (1)]
- Whenever possible children should be brought up and cared for within their own families.[s17 1(b)]
- Children should be safe and be protected by effective intervention if they are in danger.[s47 1(b)]
- When dealing with children, courts should ensure that delay is avoided.[s1 (2)]
- Children should be kept informed about what happens to them, and should participate when decisions are made about their future.[s1 (2:3a)]
- Parents continue to have parental responsibility for their children, even when their children no longer live with them. They should be kept informed about their children and participate when decisions about their children's future are made.
- Parents with children in need should be helped to bring up their children themselves. This help should be provided as a service to the child and his/her family and should be provided in partnership with the parents.

The Children Act distinguishes between:[8]

- **children in need** (section 17): those whose health and development will be significantly impaired without the provision of services
- children who are suffering, or likely to suffer **significant harm** (section 47)
- children whose **health and development is impaired** in comparison with what could reasonably be expected in a child of a similar age. This would usually be due to some form of maltreatment (section 31:10).

Where significant harm is a possibility the local authority is obliged to consider initiating enquiries to find out what is happening to the child and whether action should be taken to protect that child.

Promoting childrens' wellbeing and safeguarding them from significant harm depends crucially upon:

- effective information sharing
- working in partnership with parents
- understanding between agencies and professionals.

A further document *Framework for the Assessment of Children in Need and their Families* gives guidance to professionals and other staff involved in undertaking assessments of children and their families.[9] The framework provides a systematic way of analysing, understanding and recording what is happening to children within those families and the wider context of the community in which they live. It requires a thorough understanding of:

- the developmental needs of children
- the capacities of parents as care-givers to respond appropriately to those needs
- the impact of wider family and environmental factors on the parenting capacity and children.

The aim of the assessment process is to provide preventative and early inter-agency intervention to help reduce the extent and severity of such problems that emanate from adverse family environmental factors, such as poverty, social exclusion and other disadvantages, e.g. substance misuses by carers. An example of how this is used in relation to parental problem drug use will be discussed later in the chapter (*see* pages 96 and 98).

Developments in child protection

Following the tragic death of Victoria Climbie in 2000, the subsequent Laming report (2003) made 108 recommendations to overhaul child protection in the UK.[10] In response to this the Government published its green paper *Every Child Matters* which focused on four main areas, with proposals to:[11]

- increase support for parents and carers
- provide early intervention and effective protection
- improve accountability and integration – locally, regionally and nationally
- reform the workforce.

Also in 2004 the Government introduced into Parliament *The Children Bill* that importantly makes provision for the following.[12]

- Establishment of a children's commissioner.
- Establishment of local safeguarding children's boards (LSCBs). These are planned to be the statutory successors to Area Child Protection Committees (ACPCs), which are the current inter-agency forum for agreeing that different services and professional groups co-operate to safeguard children. Legislation will ensure that the boards should consist of representatives of councils, NHS bodies, the police, local probation boards, local prisons, young offender institutions and Child and Family Court Advisory and Support Services (CaFCaSSs).
- Establishment of children's trusts, which aim to integrate local education, social care and some health services for children and young people. A range of other local partners, such as voluntary organisations, housing and leisure services can also become involved.

Confidentiality and information sharing

Nurses working in primary care should be aware of legislation governing the disclosure of information when dealing with child protection issues. In all cases the main restrictions on disclosure of information are:

- Common law duty of confidence
- Human Rights Act
- Data Protection Act.

Guidelines for the use of these can be found in *What To Do if You're Worried a Child is Being Abused*.[13] (Summary, Appendix 1, p. 16)

It is also worth noting that through *The Children Bill* (2004) it is the Government's future intention to remove some legislative and technical barriers to better information sharing, through developing a single unique identity number and common data standards on the recording of information.[12]

Different statutory services in the context of children in need

Health

Health is a universal provision for all children including children in need. The core services start from the antenatal period and continue throughout childhood. Therefore it is often the first point of contact. It includes services for all children when they are ill, health and development surveillance for all children, and help and support for selective groups of children who are in need. Therefore each health professional has a responsibility to assess for problem drug use at the first point of contact and continue to monitor this throughout subsequent contacts.

Education

Again this is a universal provision but the point of contact is later than for health, four years of age for all children and maybe earlier for some selective groups. Education services also have a responsibility to be alert for signs of problem drug use in parents and their children, and collaborate with other agencies to ensure that children are safe.

Social services

This is not a universal provision but is accessed on a referral basis by other agencies so that child protection investigation, assessment and support (as in disability and disadvantage) can take place, and so that there is appropriate provision of other resources. Problem drug users who are parents, or about to become parents, might be referred to social services so that adequate steps are taken to safeguard children.

Health visiting principles in relation to child protection

Although the health visiting principles are over 25 years old, they remain as relevant, if not more so, than they were when they were first devised.[2] The public health role of the HV has become more high profile, at an individual, group and

Table 7.1   Principles of health visiting and child protection strategy in relation to substance misuse

Principle	Child protection	Substance misuse
Search for health needs	Awareness of child protection issues and the impact of health inequalities	Actively assess for substance misuse and be aware of the potential impact on childrens' health and wellbeing
Stimulation of the awareness of health needs	Raise parents' awareness of situations that impact on the care of their children. Alert other agencies when necessary. Map current practice and identify gaps in provision	Raise parents' awareness of how their substance misuse could be affecting the care of their children and empower them to make lifestyle changes when possible. Alert other agencies to situations where child care is compromised due to substance misuse. Map current practice and identify gaps in provision
Influence on policies affecting health	Develop strategies to review the current child protection service provided, in partnership with key agencies	Develop strategies, in collaboration with other agencies, to meet the needs of substance misusers and their children. Ensure that adequate protection is available for children in the care of problem drug users
Facilitation of health enhancing activities	Implement agreed strategies, audit changes in service and provision in collaboration with other agencies	Implement agreed strategies in relation to substance misuse. Audit changes in provision in collaboration with other agencies

community level. It is important that HVs continue to provide a universal, non-stigmatised service to all and that current financial constraints continue to allow for this. This involves an emphasis on prevention and health promotion, rather than pigeon-holing the service into a problem orientated crisis driven service, which is contrary to the whole nature of public health.

Table 7.1 indicates how the four health visiting principles can be used within child protection in relation to substance misuse.

The search for health needs
The assessment process

Health visitors need to have adequate skills in assessing parents' ability to care for their children's needs, particularly when there are early warning signs of potential factors which might compromise this ability, such as problem drug use. This assessment would involve assessing the quality of parenting, the risk to the children involved and the level of vulnerability that is present. Various models and tools have been identified to assist HVs with this process. An example of a tool which is used by HVs within one primary care trust is The Graded Care Profile.

The Graded Care Profile

The Graded Care Profile (GCP) is a tool that can be used by the HV to assess parenting and potential neglect.[14] It was developed as a practical tool to give an objective measure of the care of children across all areas of need. In the scale there are five grades based on levels of commitment to care. Parallel with the level of commitment is the degree to which a child's needs are met and this is also assessed. The basis of separation of different grades are outlined in Table 7.2.[15] (p. 1)

These grades are then applied to each of four of the areas of needs based on Maslow's hierarchy of human needs:[16]

- physical needs
- safety
- love and belonging
- esteem.

Table 7.2 Grades of levels of commitment to care

	Grade 1	Grade 2	Grade 3	Grade 4	Grade 5
1	All child's needs met	Essential needs fully met	Some essential needs unmet	Most essential needs unmet	Essential needs entirely unmet/hostile
2	Child first	Child priority	Child/carer at par	Child second	Child not considered
3	Best	Adequate	Equivocal	Poor	Worst

1 = level of care; 2 = commitment to care; 3 = quality of care.

Each area is broken down into sub-areas, for example:

- physical needs
  - nutrition
  - housing
  - clothing
  - hygiene
  - heating.

A record sheet shows all the areas and sub-areas with the five grades alongside. Rather than giving a diagnosis of neglect it defines the care showing strengths or weaknesses. As a reference point it can show changes after intervention in positive and negative directions. In practice it can be used in the following way where care of children is of concern.

- To identify care deficit where there is concern, e.g. problematic substance misuse by carers.
- Where risk appears low but care is poor it will safeguard the child by highlighting the issues. If care is good it will relieve anxiety in professionals.
- In the context of children in need it can help identify appropriate resources and target them.
- In child protection it can be used in conjunction with conventional methods in assessment of neglect and monitoring. In other forms of abuse it can be used as an adjunct in risk and need assessment.

Practitioners in primary care need to be able to use an objective measure of care across all areas of need. Tools can be helpful in this process. However, they are no substitute for professional knowledge, expertise and assessment skills, and can only ever be part of the assessment process. Appleton states that professional judgement is 'a profound element of the decision-making process in identifying vulnerability'.[17] (p. 231) Mulcahy also says that the term 'vulnerable family' is a 'dynamic, nebulous term which often defies comprehensive definition and objective measurement'.[18] (p. 257) Children of problem drug users would be deemed to be vulnerable in the eyes of any knowledgeable health professional, but the needs of children involved can vary greatly with the degree and type of problem drug use and HVs need to use all their assessment skills in order to determine whether children are in need or at risk of suffering significant harm.

In the case study below the health professional needs to consider the following points.

- What are your professional concerns?
- What are the needs of the children at this time?
- What assessments need to be made, if any?
- What do you need to tell Mike and Penny?
- What information may you need to disclose to other agencies?
- Do you know who to contact for further guidance or specialist help?
- What are your professional responsibilities?

Case study:

Mike aged 39 and Penny aged 38 are married, have twin boys (assisted pregnancy with in-vitro fertilisation) aged two years. Mike works in the City and spends many hours away from the family home. They moved into your area six months ago. You have had routine contact with the family at the Child Health Clinic. You are aware from their previous health visiting records that this is their third house move since the twin's birth.

Penny 'phones you sounding very distressed and requests help with child management issues, as she 'can't cope anymore'.

During a home visit with both parents present you notice that the house is sparsely furnished and there are few toys in evidence. You observe the twins running around the house with little structured or pretend play. They appear healthy and appropriately dressed. During discussions of child management and play strategies, they tell you that they have massive debts, have had to give up Penny's car and that they will have to move to a smaller house as the mortgage company has begun legal proceedings to repossess their home.

As you continue to listen Penny hints of relationship difficulties, and says that Mike is using most of his salary for himself. Mike admits that he has occasionally been using cocaine.

The family discussed in the case study should be classed as vulnerable due to the following factors:

- frequent house moves resulting in possible social isolation
- husband absent from the home for long periods
- debt issues
- marital problems
- behavioural problems
- possible maternal depression
- drug use problems.

The children are in need and would almost certainly benefit from access to a range of services, for example a mother and toddler group, a parenting group and support for Penny. In addition Penny and Mike might want to consider referring themselves to RELATE and the Citizen's Advice Centre for debt counselling. Discussion with Mike should take place concerning a referral to a substance misuse support and advisory service. However, the childrens' care appears to be adequate and there are no immediate concerns for their welfare. On-going support and monitoring of the situation needs to take place as there is no clear picture about the extent of Mike's drug use and the impact this may be having on the children's behavioural and developmental needs. The HV would also need to assess Penny in relation to her possible depression and support her accordingly and refer her to the GP if necessary.

Both parents need to be made aware of the potential impact of parental substance misuse on their childrens' health and development. On-going support and monitoring of the situation will be necessary to ensure that there is adequate safeguarding of the children. Clear documentation of the assessment and action plan needs to take place within the HV's records. No referral to Social Services needs to take place at this stage.

Stop here

- Think about how you can increase your assessment skills in relation to parental problem drug use, and across all age groups.
- Think about how you can increase your knowledge base in relation to problem drug use.
- How could you become more aware of services available in your local area?

Stimulation of awareness of health needs

Searching for health needs involves the HV identifying families where there are issues that impact on health and wellbeing. Once needs have been identified the HV has a responsibility to raise his/her concerns with the family and other agencies as appropriate. This section addresses situations where a significant level of concern has been raised which necessitates a referral to Social Services. Another case study is used to discuss this in relation to parental problem drug use.

Whilst research suggests that many children of problem drug users are more likely to suffer significant harm than those in the general population, it is important not to generalise or make assumptions about the impact on a child. It is vital that those working with these families understand the implications for children and complete a full assessment of the parents' ability to provide 'adequate care', as discussed in the previous section. Where there are serious concerns about the

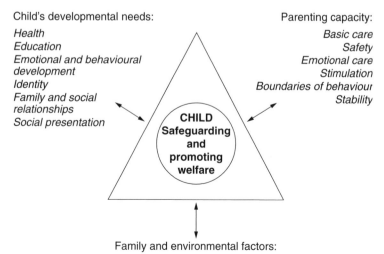

Figure 7.1   The assessment framework and process.

health and welfare of a child, a referral to Social Services will be necessary in order that a more comprehensive assessment of need is carried out. The assessment framework, as set out in the *Framework for the Assessment of Children in Need and their Families*, is the core tool for this process (*see* page 93).[9] It must be stressed that the assessment is a multi-agency task with health, education and Social Services all playing an active part, as appropriate. The HV is ideally placed to assess the child's developmental needs. Figure 7.1 illustrates the assessment framework and process.

In the case study below the health professional needs to consider the same following points.

- What are your professional concerns?
- What are the needs of the children at this time?
- What assessments need to be made, if any?
- What do you need to tell Jenny?
- What information may you need to disclose to other agencies?
- Do you know who to contact for further guidance or specialist help?
- What are your professional responsibilities?

In the case study Jenny is a vulnerable adult because she has:

- a history of heroin addiction
- a history of domestic violence
- children previously in care
- previous history of prostitution

Case study:

Jenny is 30 years of age and has spent most of her life in your area. Her mother lives locally and her father, with whom she has no contact, lives in Scotland. She has three sisters and two brothers, one of whom is on heroin. Jenny also has no contact with them.

Jenny has two children aged five and eight years. They mainly live with their father's family but also spend time with her. She has been referred to you by the Community Midwife for an antenatal assessment. During this visit Jenny tells you that she has been using heroin since she was 24. She had been in an abusive relationship and it helped ease the pain when she was beaten up. She had spent time in a refuge and stayed off heroin for eight months. Her children had been taken into care at that time. She had started using again and crack had also become a problem. At the moment she is injecting heroin into her arms about six times a week and sometimes smokes it on foil. She tells you she is using less at the moment but until recently was spending £60 a day on drugs, financed by shoplifting and prostitution. She has been in prison twice.

Jenny has a boyfriend but doesn't see him very often. She is in rented accommodation and really wants to sort her life out. She has been commenced on a methadone programme and has a key worker from the substance misuse team. She is about 16 weeks pregnant and wants to keep this baby.

- previous history of criminal convictions
- received prison sentences in the past
- a chaotic lifestyle
- her pregnancy
- an unstable relationship with her current partner
- housing needs.

The older children are at school and their father's family are the primary carers. Jenny's unborn baby may already have been exposed to the effects of heroin, whilst Jenny's lifestyle may also affect her parenting capacity in the future. She has previously had two children removed from her care. She is now on a methadone reduction programme and is requesting help from professionals. She is attending her antenatal appointments. In view of Jenny's recent history it may be considered that her unborn baby is at risk of significant harm. In order for a comprehensive assessment to take place a referral to Social Services would be necessary. A multi-agency core assessment can then take place on all the children, using the framework triangle shown in Figure 7.1, page 99.

Jenny is already receiving counselling and support from the substance misuse team. It would be important to discuss her situation with all professionals currently involved, for example the midwife, GP, school nurse and teachers at the school where her older children attend, and the substance misuse team.

It may be necessary to convene a child protection meeting, prior to the birth of the baby, to decide whether the baby needs to be placed on the child protection register and Social Services would make this decision. Jenny needs to be made aware of any risks to her current and unborn children and all referrals and decisions would need to be discussed with her so that she is able to work in partnership with the professionals.

Before any referral to Social Services takes place the HV may find it helpful to discuss Jenny's situation with a child protection specialist or manager and ensure that she has access to clinical supervision on a regular basis. Accurate and contemporaneous record keeping is essential at all times.

Stop here

- What policies and guidelines would you need to refer to nationally and locally in your area of practice?
- How would you discuss similar issues with your clients?
- Who are your local child protection contacts within the police, education and Social Services departments?
- Who would you seek professional advice and support from?

Influence on policies affecting health

Individual approaches to child protection and parental problem drug use have been discussed in earlier sections of this chapter. However HVs are also public health nurses and need to adopt a public health and community development approach to parental problem drug users as a client group. This involves influencing local and national policies which impact on local strategies and the resourcing of services. Health visitors need to take an active part in initiating and participating in steering groups that will take forward policies to safeguard local children.

'Surestart' is a government initiative which aims to achieve better outcomes for children, parents and communities by:[19]

• increased availability of childcare
• improving health, education and emotional development for young children
• supporting parents as parents and in their aspirations towards employment.

The programme is aimed at areas of disadvantage. It is predicted that 400 000 children will get access to 534 Surestart local programmes by March 2006. Health visitors take an active role within Surestart and many areas of local disadvantage also have high levels of problem drug use. This multi-agency approach to tackling inequalities in health has not yet been fully evaluated and has been criticised because of its lack of universality. However, children and families living in Surestart areas do have access to enhanced provision and resources and this can only be an advantage to those living in these areas.

Children who are removed from their parents' care due to substance misuse may become 'Looked After Children'. The present government is committed to an adoption modernisation programme and is seeking suggestions for radical ways of encouraging people to become foster carers and ensuring they are valued and recognised. Health visitors and school nurses can be in specialist roles in relation to Looked After Children and this should be encouraged.

Children's trusts are expected to be the organisational vehicle that integrate key services for children and young people under the new Director of Children's Services.[12] The trusts will bring together local authority, education and childrens' Social Services with some childrens' health services. The intention is that other services such as youth offending teams will also be involved. Children's trusts will normally be part of the local authority and will report to locally elected members. Health visitors could become change agents in these new trusts and in the case of problem drug use could influence the way that services are provided and resourced to meet the needs of this client group.

Health visitors need to actively look for opportunities to enhance the care of clients, client groups and communities, whether in relation to problem drug use or in relation to other areas of health need. This is a dynamic time in health and social care and HVs need to be ready to seize the challenge of these changing times.

Stop here

• How do you have an influence on local policies?
• Do you feel that you could take a more active part in influencing national policy, perhaps by responding to consultation papers prior to policies being agreed?
• Can you identify any gaps in service provision locally?

Facilitation of health enhancing activities

Health visitors need to become actively involved with auditing service provision and where gaps exist collaborate with local communities and other agencies to introduce innovative ways of working. It is essential that local communities are involved in identifying needs in their locality and successful community development initiatives always involve active participation, and often leadership, from residents who live in the area. Health visitors can become facilitators and encourage clients to lead initiatives to improve services locally. They can also respond to needs by providing individual, group and community-wide health promotional programmes. Local residents are often very upset by problem drug use in their area and are concerned about their children abusing drugs or alcohol. They also might be concerned about the care of children locally if they are in the care of problem drug users. Health visitors can often empower individuals and communities to bring about change and this needs to be an important part of their role.

Brocklehurst *et al.* discuss a home visiting programme which is designed to support vulnerable children and their families.[20] This programme aims to improve child and maternal health and wellbeing following identification of vulnerability at the antenatal booking-in clinic. The home visiting continues from the second trimester of pregnancy until 12 months after the baby is born. These mothers are visited weekly by a specially trained health visitor and a problem based partnership approach is taken. The full evaluation has not yet taken place but results could be encouraging in helping to break the cycle of deprivation and abuse. However, this approach is time-consuming and potentially very stressful for the HV and very resource heavy for the health visiting service. The extent to which the benefits outweigh the resource issues will be important to assess, and services planned on lessons learnt could make a real difference to child protection and parental problem drug use for those who have access to such programmes.

Stop here

- Can you identify any community development projects locally which could be perceived as helping to safeguard children?
- If so, what approaches are they using?
- Are you aware of any means of auditing these initiatives?
- How would this fit in the clinical governance agenda of your local Primary Care Trust?
- How are the needs of vulnerable families in your area addressed?
- Do you think that intensive visiting programmes are the way forward?

Checklist of issues

- The welfare of the child is paramount.
- Accurate and contemporaneous record keeping is essential in all child protection cases.
- Problem drug use needs to be actively searched for.

- Assessment is key to identifying children in need.
- Children of parental problem drug users are potentially at risk of suffering significant harm.
- Multi-agency working is essential in all cases of child protection.
- Mandatory training in child protection should be accessed by all health and social care personnel who come into contact with children.
- Clinical supervision should be available to all who work within child protection.
- All HVs need to be aware of their accountability and responsibility in relation to child protection.
- Inequalities in health are strong influencing factors in the health and wellbeing of individuals and communities.
- Cultural and religious influences should be taken into account when appropriate but these should not override the welfare of a child.

Summary

Health visitors are ideally placed within the community to search for health needs where there are issues in relation to problem drug use. Using their assessment skills they can identify where on the continuum of vulnerability childrens' needs lie. They are able to stimulate the awareness of health needs by raising parental awareness and referral to other agencies. They can also map current practice and identify gaps in service provision. Their role in influencing policies affecting health is to develop strategies to review current child protection services in collaboration with other agencies. These are all developments of health enhancing activities as well as empowering individuals and communities to become actively involved in improving the outcome for all children. Problem drug use is endemic and is an increasing area of health need and one that will continue to challenge all those who work within the primary healthcare setting.

Documents such as *The National Service Framework for Children, Young People and Maternity Services* and *The Children Bill* (2004) continue to provide measures to safeguard all children.[12,21]

References

1   Harbin F and Murphy M (eds) (2000) *Substance Misuse and Child Care*. Russell House Publishing Ltd, Dorset.
2   Council for Education and Training of Health Visitors (1977) *An Investigation into the Principles of Health Visiting*. CETHV, London.
3   Advisory Council on the Misuse of Drugs (2003) *Hidden Harm: responding to the needs of children of problem drug users*. Home Office, London. www.drugs.gov.uk/ReportsandPublications/NationalStrategy/1054733801/hidden_harm.pdf
4   Lilias A (2000) What are the risks to children of parental substance misuse? In: F Harbin and M Murphy (eds) *Substance Misuse and Child Care*. Russell House Publishing Ltd, Dorset.
5   Department of Health, Home Office and Department for Education and Employment (1999) *Working Together to Safeguard Children: a guide to inter-agency working to safeguard and promote the welfare of children*. HMSO, London.

6 Savage M (1993) Can early indicators of neglecting families be observed: a comparative study of neglecting and non-neglecting families. Unpublished dissertation. University of Ulster, Belfast. In: D Iwaniec (1995) *The Emotionally Abused and Neglected Child: identification, assessment and intervention.* John Wiley and Sons, Chichester.

7 Browne K, Hanks H, Stratton P *et al.* (2002) *Early Prediction and Prevention of Child Abuse: a handbook.* John Wiley and Sons, Chichester.

8 Department of Health (1991) *The Children Act 1989.* HMSO, London.

9 Department of Health (2000) *Framework for the Assessment of Children in Need and their Families.* HMSO, London.

10 Lord Laming (2003) *The Victoria Climbié Inquiry.* HMSO, London.

11 Department for Education and Skills (2004) *Every Child Matters: next steps.* DfES Publications, Nottingham.

12 House of Lords (2004) *The Children Bill.* HMSO, London.

13 Department of Health (2003) *What To Do if You're Worried a Child is Being Abused.* Department of Health, London. www.doh.gov.uk/safeguarding children/index.htm

14 Srivastava O and Polnay L (1997) Field trial of Graded Care Profile (GPC) scale: a new measure of care. *Archives of Disease in Childhood.* **76**: 337–40.

15 Srivastava O (1995) *Graded Care Profile Scale: a qualitative scale for measure of care of children.* Luton Area Child Protection Committee, Luton, Bedfordshire.

16 Maslow A (1954) *Motivation and Personality.* Harper and Row, New York.

17 Appleton J (1995) Health visitor assessment of vulnerability. *Health Visitor.* **68**: 228–31.

18 Mulcahy H (2004) 'Vulnerable family' as understood by public health nurses. *Community Practitioner.* **77**(7): 257–60.

19 www.surestart.gov.uk

20 Brocklehurst N, Barlow J, Kirkpatrick S *et al.* (2004) The contribution of health visitors to supporting vulnerable children and their families at home. *Community Practitioner.* **77**(5): 175–9.

21 Department of Health (2004) *The National Service Framework for Children, Young People and Maternity Services.* HMSO, London. www.dh.gov.uk/Policy AndGuidance/HealthAndSocialCareTopics/Childrens/fr/en

CHAPTER 8

Treatment and its effectiveness in relapse prevention associated with crack cocaine

Aidan Gray

Before beginning any significant work with crack cocaine users it is important for practitioners to examine what barriers to effective treatment may exist within their service. If the policy, practice and knowledge of the service is embedded in treating opiate users then barriers to effective treatment of crack cocaine users will probably be present.

Stereotypes

One of the biggest barriers to treatment for crack cocaine users has been the undeniably strong stereotypes associated with crack use. These stereotypes are most commonly rooted in historical racism, attitudes to poverty and the fear that these issues bring when associated with inaccurate and sensationalist reporting by the media. The power of these stereotypes should not be underestimated when examining treatment options as they not only influence commissioners and treatment providers (therefore practice and policy), they also affect the users themselves. Although the origins of crack users' extremely negative stereotypes can be traced as far back as the mid 1500s with Spain's conquest of the Incan civilisation, its modern image was primarily formed in the early 1900s in the USA.

In 1901 the Senate adopted a resolution that forbade the sale by American traders of opium and alcohol 'to aboriginal tribes and uncivilized races'. These provisions were later extended to include 'uncivilized elements in America itself and in its territories, such as Indians, Alaskans, and the inhabitants of Hawaii, railroad workers, and immigrants at ports of entry'. With alcohol and opium being prohibited to the Black community, cocaine was one of the few options left. This selective prohibition led to a general increase in the use of cocaine and also in some cases replaced the use of alcohol as uncovered by the *British Medical Journal* in 1902.[1]

> On many of the Yazoo plantations this year the Negroes refused to work unless they could be assured that there was some place in the

neighbourhood where they could get cocaine, and it is said that some planters kept the drug in stock among plantation supplies, and issued regular rations of cocaine just as they used to issue rations of whisky.

Colonel Watson (a well known anti-cocaine campaigner) not only linked the use of cocaine to the Black community but also linked madness and criminal behaviour with its use as well.[1]

Unquestionably the drug rapidly affects the brain and the result has been that, in the South, the asylums for the insane are overflowing with the unfortunate victims.

He went on to conclude that:

Many of the horrible crimes committed in the Southern States by the colored people can be traced back directly to the cocaine habit.

In the *New York Times* in 1914, Dr Edward H Williams commented under the headline 'Negro Cocaine "Fiends" are a new Southern Menace'; that:

Since this gruesome evidence is supported by the printed records of insane hospitals, police courts, jails and penitentiaries, there is no escaping the conviction that drug taking has become a race menace in certain regions south of the line.[1]

It can be easy to dismiss attitudes that were held 100 years ago as being uninformed and a symptom of less enlightened times, however these attitudes still persist today in what can be termed as 'politically correct' language.

In 1989 Robert Stutman a senior Drug Enforcement Agent addressed the Ninth Annual Drugs Conference of Assistant Chief Police Officers in Wales and proceeded to continue the manipulation of facts regarding crack that he had helped develop in the USA.[2] He introduced the idea (to the UK) that after three hits of crack '75 per cent will become physically addicted' and went on to describe the 'crack epidemic' phenomena as 'no other drug in history comes close to spreading that quickly'. Parents were targeted by his suggestion that if he 'wanted to design a drug that's aimed for kids', he 'couldn't improve on it [crack]' and he played on the fear of violence by describing the change of guns issued to all agents in the Drug Enforcement Agency (DEA) from a .38 handgun to sub-machine guns, and stating 'That is what has happened in one country basically because of crack'.

And finally he discussed the issue of race:

Right now crack is controlled by a fairly large number of organisations, basically because of its background: Dominicans and Jamaicans ... now again, I don't have to tell any of you gentlemen this, but you have a large number of Jamaicans in this country.[2]

In 1992 Robert Stutman revealed in his autobiography *Dead on Delivery* that:

There was no doubt in my mind that crack was on its way to becoming a national problem. But, to speed up the process of convincing

Washington, I needed to make it a national issue and quickly. I began a lobbying effort and I used the media. Reporters were only too willing to co-operate ...[1]

The development of policy on stereotypes can be seen in the Government's action on demand reduction in the UK where they have seemingly concentrated upon cocaine importation from Jamaica. In 2004 an article in the *Guardian* reported under the headline 'Jamaican Cocaine Mules Reined In' that:

Customs claimed success in its two-year operation to stem the flow of cocaine smugglers from Jamaica yesterday. New figures show the number of cocaine-swallowing 'mules' detected on arrival has fallen sharply, from a high of 730 in the year to June 2002, to 185 in the year to June 2003, to only 41 in the past 12 months.[3]

Before this operation began approximately 7% of cocaine importation was via Jamaica (probably less now) yet the vast majority of cocaine being imported into this country is via Europe (approximately 65%).

Stop here

It is vital that all treatment services understand from where the stereotypes for crack use have developed and that there is an awareness of this when developing services or providing treatment.

Opiate-dominant service provision

Crack cocaine is a different drug when compared to opiates (almost the entire opposite) and services need to acknowledge that over the last 20 years national policies and practice have predominately reflected the needs of opiate users leading to imbalances in provision within generic treatment providers. As early as 1995 UK research on crack and cocaine use identified that crack users where not accessing services because they were too opiate orientated.[4] Subsequent studies have highlighted similar problems and with the recent trend in heroin and crack combination use, have also identified that opiate users already engaged with treatment services are only accessing for their heroin use.

There is a growing argument for not developing specific crack services as there has been a recent increase in the number of traditionally primary heroin users taking crack. However what is not usually acknowledged is that UK treatment services are dominated by opiate treatment at a time when the main drugs used in the UK are stimulants. Maybe the argument would be better placed to quite simply say:

'Generic services should become truly generic.'

And be able to work effectively with the whole range of drugs currently being used in the UK at the moment.

> **Stop here**
>
> Examine practice and policies within your agencies to ascertain whether they are appropriate and effective for crack cocaine users.

Understand how crack affects users

The dominance of opiates within the UK drug field has also led to an imbalance in the knowledge of other drugs. This is particularly acute when examining the issue of crack cocaine treatment and has sometimes led to practitioners describing heroin withdrawals to primary crack users. This does not build confidence in drug services.

If you are going to work with crack and cocaine it is imperative that you understand the drug with which you are engaged. All engines work on similar principles, however if you have only been trained on petrol engines, diesel engines could be a little tricky.

Understanding crack and cocaine is essential in the development of service provision and individual treatment patterns. As a basic requirement practitioners should understand:

- how crack works as a drug
- potential physical and mental health problems arising from its use.

Understanding of a drug not only aids treatment development and provision but it can also be utilised as a useful tool in the development of a trusting relationship and the continued engagement in services.[5]

How crack cocaine works

The first thing to say about crack and cocaine is that it does not produce a physical dependence in the way that we understand heroin dependence. It can, however, create a very strong psychological dependence. Crack and cocaine work by triggering the release of chemicals that are already present in the body. It is important to note that these chemicals are part of the body's response to danger and pleasure.

Adrenaline
Adrenaline is normally released as part of a response to danger or excitement and heightens the senses and enables the body to work at peak performance. It does this by:

- **increasing heart rate**: this is to increase the blood flow around the body, which also increases the speed at which oxygen reaches the muscles
- **increasing breathing rate**: short and shallow breaths increase the amount of oxygen in the bloodstream

- **butterflies in the stomach**: this is due to blood leaving the stomach and being diverted to the arms and legs where it is most needed
- **sweating**: the body is getting hotter and sweating is the body's cooling system.

Users may recognise the above symptoms as the feelings they get when they are craving for crack/cocaine or are just about to score. When they do use crack they are again releasing adrenaline because of cocaine's effects on noradrenaline and the adrenal system. The persistent release of adrenaline caused by cocaine use can lead to decreased need for sleep, loss of appetite, visual and auditory hallucinations, impaired cognitive ability (due to lack of sleep), severe anxiety and paranoia. The environment that the drug is used in and the mind set of the user will also contribute to the intensity of the highs and severity of the lows experienced. For instance if people use in a hostile environment like a crack house or with someone they don't trust then the feelings of anxiety and paranoia can be worse.

Dopamine

The 'high' experienced by a person taking crack or cocaine is produced by a chemical called dopamine. Cocaine changes the way the brain works by changing the way the nerve cells (neurones) communicate with each other. Nerve cells in the brain normally send messages to each other using chemicals called neurotransmitters. These neurotransmitters fire across a gap between each cell and attach on to receptor sites. Once the message has been received a transporting cell mops up the neurotransmitter so that the levels in these chemicals remain balanced.

Dopamine is a neurotransmitter that helps produce the feelings of pleasure and is released by the use of cocaine. Cocaine works by simply blocking the transporting cell causing a build up of dopamine at the receptor sites. This leads to the extended feelings of pleasure that are experienced when taking cocaine and also ultimately leads to the 'downs' experienced by causing depletion in these chemicals because they can't get back. Imagine getting a brand new credit card, you have extended spending power for a period of time, you have fun and then the bill arrives through your letterbox.

'Chasing that high' is a lost cause because the more that people use the more blocks are put in place and the less dopamine they have. After a user's first hit they will be on a downward spiral chasing a high that is impossible to get. The depletion of dopamine is partly responsible for the 'come down' or 'crash', making users feel bad and reinforcing the need for another hit, then another and another, etc. Depletion in these neurotransmitters can also cause a chemical depression, which can sometimes combine with other life events (loss of job, partner, etc.) and possibly lead to suicidal thoughts. Depletion can also lead to some users experiencing severe mood changes.

Combination

The combination of increased adrenaline levels and low dopamine levels after a period of using can produce the feelings of being 'wired' or 'prang'. Users may at this stage opt for a 'downer' drug like alcohol, cannabis or heroin to help them cope with this feeling. What they are doing is suppressing the effect of the adrenaline, which sometimes makes it easier to 'come down' from crack or cocaine. Box 8.1 can be used with clients to help explain how crack and cocaine work.

Box 8.1   How crack and cocaine work

Adrenaline (noradrenaline)
Initial release: (craving, anticipation)
Danger and excitement

- increased heart rate
- faster breathing
- sweating
- shaking/can't stay still
- butterflies/sickness in stomach

Prolonged release: (continued use can cause the following)

- can't sleep
- don't want to eat
- increased anxiety ('wired' or 'prang')
- harder to think clearly
- hallucinations (also interactions with brain chemicals)
- paranoia

Dopamine and serotonin
Initial release: (first high/buzz)
Reward and reinforcement

- very strong first high
- feelings of confidence
- euphoric/orgasmic
- compulsion to use again

Prolonged release: (depletion of dopamine)

- repeated compulsion to use
- buzz getting shorter and lower
- comedown or 'crash'
- loss of interest in things not related to cocaine
- mood swings
- depression

Cravings and compulsion to use

The urge to use crack or cocaine comes from a combination of the effects of adrenaline and dopamine. To begin with adrenaline is usually released by a 'trigger' (something that users associate with crack or cocaine), such as meeting someone they use with, emotional feelings or getting the money to use. This causes the symptoms described above (initial adrenaline release) and quickly they can be on a 'mission' to use, feel agitated or anticipation at the thought of using. However, when they have used once the compulsion to use is created by dopamine. Dopamine works within the primitive areas of the brain and is partly responsible for the drive that we experience to seek food and have sex, etc. Taking crack or cocaine exaggerates this drive and reinforces drug seeking behaviour leading to continued use of the drug even when users know that the 'high' cannot be reached again.[6]

Crack/cocaine and health

Crack and cocaine can damage users' health in many ways and in some instances these can be fatal. Some of these risks can be increased by the way that they use (larger amounts, binge use and combinations of drugs like alcohol, heroin, etc.) and also by the route of use. The bottom line is that there is no safe way to use. Some of the health problems that can be caused by crack and cocaine use include:[6]

- cardiovascular problems and failure
- respiratory problems

- strokes and intracranial haemorrhaging
- brain seizures
- liver damage (especially in conjunction with alcohol)
- kidney damage
- complications with pregnancy (although many US studies have subsequently be shown to be flawed or overblown)
- complications with existing psychiatric disorders (ADHD, bi-polar disorder, depression, schizophrenia)
- excited delirium/cocaine psychosis
- chemically induced depression (dopamine and serotonin depletion)
- impaired immune system
- severe weight loss
- bloodborne viruses
- complications associated with route of use such as:
  - 'crack lung'
  - pulmonary haemorrhage
  - deep vein thrombosis (DVT)
  - increased occurrence of abscesses
- general poor health associated with drug using lifestyle.

Stop here

All services and practitioners wanting to engage crack cocaine users in treatment should understand how the drug works and possible health complications. This knowledge should be built into the development of services and treatment plans.

Understanding local need

In looking to provide effective treatment for crack cocaine users, services providers should be clear about the following.

Crack cocaine users already attracted into the services

In many parts of the UK crack and heroin markets are now beginning to merge, with heroin dealers selling crack, and crack dealers selling heroin. One of the major consequences of this is that many primary heroin users are now using crack cocaine.[7,8] Although the majority of this user group is accessing services for advice, information, needle exchanges, etc. they may not be raising the issue of crack use or be underplaying its significance. Examine the cost of their crack use against heroin, the developing physical and mental health consequences and how crack use has had an impact on their overall drug use so that the true effect of crack cocaine use can be weighed against planned treatment options.

> **Stop here**
>
> Be aware that you may already be working with a significant amount of crack cocaine users. Examine assessment protocol to ensure that crack is being asked about appropriately to help develop awareness of an existing crack client group.

Crack cocaine users not attracted into the services

Although many services are attracting existing clients that are beginning to use crack cocaine or may consider it to be secondary use, there will probably be a significant proportion of primary crack users that is just not accessing services at all. As mentioned previously in this chapter many primary crack users view drug treatment services as being for heroin users, so what is the point of accessing them? If you want to attract primary crack users into your service and also make crack/heroin users more aware of treatment options then advertise them including the words 'crack' or 'cocaine' to avoid misunderstanding. Ultimately the best way to attract users into your service is by word of mouth.

To do this effectively you will need to deliver a service that crack users feel is useful and orientated towards their needs. Saying that you offer a service and then not providing any treatment options orientated towards crack cocaine will have the opposite effect.

In attracting users into services, thought should also be given to crack cocaine users who do not want to stop using. Most crack specific services focus on abstinence as the primary goal. Consequently there has been little focus on areas such as harm reduction or controlled use. If services are aiming to attract current users, the service developed should reflect the needs of the client group.

> **Stop here**
>
> Offer services that are appropriate to the users you want to attract and if you say that you are working with crack cocaine users make sure that you do.

Types of services that may need to be provided

There are many types of service/treatment that can be developed or re-orientated for crack cocaine users. Some of the treatment examples that can be found in the UK include:

- specific user groups/unions
- harm reduction initiatives
- outreach
- crisis intervention centres
- primary care interventions

- drop-in services
- weekly groups
- structured day programmes
- residential services.

Agencies may want to develop specific services for crack cocaine users or re-orientate existing services towards crack cocaine.

Stop here

Be aware of the range of services that can be delivered for crack cocaine users and existing services can also be re-orientated towards crack rather than developing completely separate services.

Types of services that can realistically be provided

To do this effectively services may want to conduct a local/project-led needs analysis. Needs assessments are only as good as the questions that you ask and if you do not ask the right questions from the start the then information that you collate may not help you develop the best service. For example, if you are working with an increasingly high number of injecting crack and heroin users and do not ask about the possible increase in hits per day you may not be offering clients enough clean needles and increase the chances of sharing or using contaminated 'works'.

Undertaking an analysis will also help your service to make decisions regarding the best use of resources set against the identified needs, help you place crack orientated services within a generic framework and plan the appropriate use of what can realistically be very limited budgets.

Stop here

Look at conducting local or project needs assessments so that informed decisions can be made in relation to services development.

Effective services provision

For services providers to have a better understanding of the needs of crack cocaine users in their area they should look at the following.

Advice and information

Whatever the level of service you decide to provide one of the most important aspects will be to educate users around crack and cocaine and in particular how it works. This can help to build up:

- client's knowledge of crack, its use and possible dangers
- a better understanding of potential services and their benefits
- trust with the worker/agency.

Health treatment

Because crack cocaine treatment is getting its impetus from the criminal justice agenda it can be very easy to miss or minimise the appropriate levels of healthcare. There is a wider range of health issues associated with crack cocaine than there is with heroin so it is vitally important that all services (especially those offering initial contact points) provide crack orientated health assessments.

Users themselves may also not be aware of the full extent of their health problems as they may have been masked by drug use or in some cases the anaesthetic properties of crack again reinforcing the need for appropriate health checks.

Harm reduction

Crack cocaine use can be associated with high levels of health complaints, drug related deaths and also an increase in criminal involvement.[9] It is therefore important to consider specific harm reduction interventions when developing treatment services that are engaging users who want to continue to use.

Harm reduction for crack users usually rests in a political grey region which has led to a historic underdevelopment in this area. However, at the same time as there has been a reluctance to embrace crack orientated/specific harm reduction there has been a 50% increase in UK cocaine related deaths. Harm reduction initiatives should be considered for the three primary routes of use (snorting, smoking and injecting) and clear protocols developed within statutory and voluntary service provision. Users will also need to be educated around harm reduction to bring the levels of knowledge about crack and cocaine up to that of heroin.

Abstinence based treatment

Abstinence based treatment does offer the opportunity to increase the amount of information given to clients and build upon foundation information such as:

- how crack works
- health implications
- harm reduction.

Within a short period of time of stopping the use of crack cocaine clients will be able to concentrate for longer periods of time, have less anxiety/paranoia and feel less depressed. This will be due to brain and body chemistry beginning to rebalance, essentially leading to the ability to work at a higher level.

Once clients reach this level then services have the ability to begin to build their knowledge around various aspects of the client's drug use. Treatment sessions should include the following foundation areas.

Triggers

It is important for a client to understand how triggers work, how this links in with the 'fight and flight' response and what *their* main triggers are. Users can often use the same set of triggers over and over again unless awareness is gained. Further information and knowledge can also be gained through the examination of lapse and relapse. Work with clients to identify what their main triggers are and then develop strategies to avoid, change or minimise them.

Cravings

Triggers usually lead to cravings, so again it is important for users to understand what they are, the types of craving associated with crack cocaine and what to do when cravings start. Users often feel powerless with craving and knowledge can change their ability to take control of craving situations.

There are two main things to remember when dealing with cravings:

- they always need a trigger (face, place, money, etc.)
- they are not a need, they are a *want*.

Cravings associated with crack cocaine are usually a combination of physical, chemical and emotional factors.

- Physical feelings of sweating, heart beating faster, butterflies in the stomach, anxiety and increased breathing rate come from the release of adrenaline into the system triggering off the 'flight' or 'fight' response.
- Compulsion to use, single minded behaviour and a belief that a client needs the drug come from the reward and reinforcing effects of dopamine and serotonin.
- Emotional factors like depression, celebration, boredom and isolation can provide justifications to use and also contribute to irrational thinking.

Because of the strong connection between the fight and flight response and craving it is important to look at other situations that might trigger the response normally as these situations can be misinterpreted as cravings. These situations may include feeling anxious about:

- receiving dental treatment
- starting college or a new job
- going for an interview
- family reunions.

Euphoric recall

Changing your life is a very difficult thing to do and at some points it is natural to look back. In doing this it is usually the good or exciting times that are focused upon and this increases the chance of developing cravings.

The reality of euphoric recall is a bit like a movie trailer, full of excitement and action but never gets the reality of the film across. Giving understanding of what euphoric recall is and how it can lead to craving situations can help prepare the client for when they happen. Doing exercises that look at the pro's and con's of drugs are useful at this stage as this can help identify the reality of the client's drug use and in effect show the whole film and not just the highlights.

Prevention strategies

Concentrate upon strategies to help clients keep safe and avoid situations that may lead to use. Make these realistic, practical and achievable. Enabling a client to understand their patterns of use can form a starting point for treatment/understanding. The patterns of use handout can be utilised and strategies developed that are pertinent to the user such as the following.[10]

- Avoid people, places and faces. Work out routes that take you safely past areas or keep to areas that don't have associations.
- Carry envelopes with name, address and stamp. Too much money? Starting to crave? Post it to yourself. You get the money in the morning or next day and have time to think what to do with it.
- Carry relaxing oils. Sniff in times of crisis.
- Don't carry more than £5, £10, and £15; whatever amount triggers you off.
- Inform people (safely) that you don't use anymore. Don't leave doors open.
- Get rid of all paraphernalia (and don't go shopping the next day to buy foil, bottles of water, and a packet of Blu Tak to put the new posters up with!).
- Plan ahead. See if dangerous situations can be identified.
- Plan support for dangerous situations.
- Always have a plan 'B'. Where can I run to when I need to be safe?
- Build alternative support networks: Narcotics Anonymous, college, clean friends, hobbies, etc.
- Use alternative therapies/breathing exercises to help reduce craving.

Some research suggests that when working with severe problems the length of time in treatment should be considered proportionally as this can help improve overall treatment outcomes; those treated for 90 days or longer had the best outcomes.[11]

Lapse and relapse

Usually the process of stopping the use of drugs will involve lapses that can sometimes lead to full relapses. It is therefore vitally important to work with lapses quickly and effectively.

The process of lapse and relapse can sometimes be difficult to quantify, the following definitions can be used as a guide.

- **Abstained**: Clients who, once they enter into treatment, do not use crack or cocaine again.
- **Lapse**: Clients who may experience short-term (one to ten days) return(s) to use, followed by longer periods of abstinence.
- **Extended lapse**: Clients who experience an extended period of use (two to 12 weeks) but have maintained contact with treatment services and follow this use with long periods of abstinence.
- **Full relapse**: Clients who experience a full return to drug use after a period of treatment and are choosing not to engage in services.

Lapse management

A lapse does not mean that clients have gone back to square one. If they don't work with the incident then they may miss the opportunity to learn from mistakes, make the same mistake again or continue on the path to a full relapse.

Clients need to understand:

* what happened.
* how it happened.
* how they can stop it happening again.

Start by tracing the events that led to the client using. They may need to go over things a few times going one step further back each time to trace their initial 'set up'. Ask who they were with. How did they feel emotionally/physically? Where did they get the money from? What justifications were used?

Extended lapse management

Some lapses will extend past a few days of use and can either move into a full relapse or, on occasions, develop into an extended lapse. Although use may be chaotic again, the willingness to continue treatment is what differentiates this from a full relapse.

Full relapse

Some clients will return to their previous levels of use and usually disengage from structured services. If they re-engage with treatment services the treatment options offered will usually reflect those of a new referral, however the initial lapse that led to the full relapse can be examined so that knowledge can be gained from the experience.

Aftercare

Aftercare can encompass a range of support for a longer period of time to enable a client to reintegrate into society. Clients also need quick access to a service if they have a lapse, irrespective of how long ago they left treatment. Clients need to be reassured that they do not have to wait until they have experienced a full-blown relapse before re-engaging. Having the ability to seek help at times of vulnerability or crisis could be crucial in averting relapse.

Agencies should be able to work with lapse or potential lapse quickly and when the client needs it. If a client has been drug free for a number of years and had a lapse they may still be in employment or education, their relationship will probably be intact and their financial situation should not have deteriorated to the point of needing major input. A quick response can mean the difference between a lapse and the agency having to begin work again with a full relapse.

Summary

Working with crack and cocaine users does not mean that there are completely new areas of work to be addressed, nor does it mean learning a completely new set of skills.[12] However, developing good knowledge of crack cocaine and understanding related issues are essential if users are to be offered effective treatment.

References

1   Streatfield D (2001) *Cocaine: an unauthorised biography*. Virgin Publishing Ltd, London.

2   Stutman R (1989) *Transcript of speech to the ACPOW.* Drugscope Library, London.

3   Travis A (2004) Jamaican cocaine mules reined in. *The Guardian.* 7 July.

4   Donnall M, Seivewright N, Douglas J and Draycott T (1995) *National Cocaine Treatment Study: the effectiveness of treatments offered to cocaine/crack users.* University of Manchester Drug Misuse Unit and Community Health Sheffield NHS Trust.

5   National Treatment Agency (2002) *Drug Services Briefing: treating cocaine/crack dependence.* Department of Health, London.

6   Gray A and D'Agostino T (2003) *Crack and Cocaine Information Pack.* COCA, London.

7   Gray A, Sangster D, D'Agostino T and Reid R (2004) *Crack in Leeds 2004: Needs Analysis.* COCA, London.

8   Ward J, Mattick RP and Hall W (1998) *Methadone Maintainence Treatment and Other Opioid Replacement Therapies.* Harwood Academic Publishers, Reading.

9   Simpson DD, Joe GW, Fletcher BW *et al.* (1999) A national evaluation of treatment outcomes for cocaine dependence. *Archives of General Psychiatry.* **56**: 507–14.

10   Gray A (2002) *Treating Crack or Cocaine Misuse: a resource pack for treatment providers.* NTA, London.

11   Laranjeira R, Rassi R, Dunn J *et al.* (2001) Crack cocaine – a two-year follow-up of treated patients. *Journal of Addictive Diseases.* **20**(1).

12   National Treatment Agency (2002) *Commissioning Cocaine/Crack Treatment.* Department of Health, London.

Further reading

• Ford C (2004) *Guidance for Working with Cocaine and Crack Users in Primary Care.* RCGP, London.

CHAPTER 9

The role of the practice counsellor in substance misuse treatments

Sue Gardner

Introduction

This chapter examines the part played by 'talking treatments' in providing a range of services to people who misuse drugs and/or alcohol. The field of talking treatments involves confusing terminology and several different names for what can seem like similar approaches. Interchangeable generic terms include 'psychological therapy', 'psychological treatments', 'talking therapies' and 'talking treatments'. Within the field there are two main traditions, psychotherapy and counselling which are briefly described in this chapter. Some forms of talking treatments have been particularly useful in substance misuse and these are also described. The term 'structured counselling' is specifically used by the National Treatment Agency (NTA) and its definition is outlined. The reasons for some people requiring talking treatments are examined as is the evidence for the efficacy of these approaches. The role of the practice counsellor is briefly described. Finally there is a 'toolkit' of useful techniques to enhance the work of all primary care staff.

Throughout the chapter 'client' is used instead of patient or service user as this is the term traditionally used in a talking treatment context. Also, given that the key psychological issues in substance misuse are motivation and behaviour change the type of substance being misused (drugs or alcohol or both) is of less importance than the meaning of the misuse.

What are psychotherapy and counselling?

The most recent and comprehensive attempt to answer this question came from the Department of Health:[1]

> In essence, different forms of psychotherapy have evolved to offer remediation of mental health problems and symptoms by structured interventions. Different forms of counselling emphasise the individual's resources, rather than psychopathology, with a focus on a reflective, experiential process. Here the patient's concerns are rephrased and clarified in order that he or she may develop a greater sense of wellbeing

and cope with life difficulties differently. There is emphasis on mental health promotion rather than 'treating disorders'. Historically, as this approach developed outside the NHS, and it was applied later to medical settings, counselling tended to be briefer and counsellors worked with patients who were less ill.

The terminological confusion is exacerbated by the common practice of denoting all psychological therapy delivered in primary care as 'counselling'. In fact, a number of 'counsellors' employed in primary care are qualified psychotherapists.

Talking treatments are often organised in a 'tiered' way, where the amount of expert help applied is in response to varying degrees of need. This is now common practice in a wide range of health settings.

For psychological therapies a tiered approach is likely to involve the following six stages.

1 **Bibliotherapy**: The provision of leaflets and books that might give people practical advice on how to help themselves.
2 **Advice**: Someone with knowledge and experience giving people help tailored to suit the individual and their situation.
3 **Brief problem solving and support**: Someone, again with knowledge and experience, being able to help people identify their specific problems and ways in which these problems might be tackled, either by the individual or by others.
4 **Counselling**: In primary care this is provided by a wide range of health professionals including nurses, HVs, community psychiatric nurses, psychologists and GPs who have had special training. There are also counsellors who did not have a health background before their counselling or psychotherapy training. Professional organisations such as the British Association for Counselling and Psychotherapy (BACP) recommend a minimum of a diploma course (450 hours of training including skills and theory) and considerable supervised practice.
5 **Structured groups**: These are for people often whose lives and day-to-day functioning are impaired by mental health problems. Groups usually have a specific problem or issue that they focus on. The benefits of a group include hearing from others about their problems and discussing new solutions. The feelings of loneliness, guilt and inadequacy that many people have can be reduced by sharing these feelings with others.

Groups require skilled facilitators, careful planning and a clear structure. Care must be taken to ensure that every group member is encouraged to contribute, that no one person dominates the meeting and that discussions are constructive.
6 **Formal psychotherapy**: This category includes four main types:
   – psychodynamic psychotherapy
   – cognitive behavioural therapy
   – cognitive analytic therapy
   – systemic or family therapy

These psychotherapies require specialised training and are briefly described on pages 128–30.

What is structured counselling?

The NTA's *Models of Care* describe structured counselling as a skilled activity with:

> Assessment, clearly defined treatment plans and treatment goals and regular reviews, as opposed to advice and information, drop-in support and informed key working.

> ... which must be provided by competent and accredited counsellors. Service providers will utilise counselling skills within their practice, but this should not be equated with the provision of structured care planned counselling.[2]

Structured counselling can therefore be either psychotherapy or counselling as applied in substance misuse. Some talking therapies are 'approaches' or a set of principles to guide a practitioner into interacting with a client. Other, formal therapies have a more comprehensive theoretical framework and a systematic set of approaches. In reality many skilled practitioners have been trained in several approaches and theoretical frameworks and will apply the 'tools' that best suit the needs of the client they are trying to help.

Why do some clients need structured counselling?

Most people accessing services have a range of emotions including:

- anxiety – uncertainty about the future
- depression – relating to the loss of recreational, enjoyable substance misuse
- grief – that the substance misuse might have to stop
- anger – that a pleasurable activity has turned into pain
- low self-esteem – feeling that they have 'failed' to control their substance use.

By using empathic, interpersonal skills as part of the treatment, these emotions will be resolved by the client receiving a respectful service. For some people, however, these issues may have been present before the substance misuse began or may have been exacerbated by the misuse, and structured counselling will be helpful in untangling the different emotions and helping in their resolution.

There are certain protective factors that seem to help clients either by reducing the effect of the substance misuse or by speeding their recovery. These include:

- having a sense of self-esteem
- having some experiences of safety and affection as a child
- some supportive relationships
- some recognisable skills and abilities.

Those clients who have more difficulties include those:

- whose early childhood experiences were abusive in some way
- who are already overloaded in terms of life stress

- who have mental health problems
- who do not have confidence in their ability to cope
- to whom all of the above apply.

It is becoming clearer, however, that the majority of people who change from substance misuse do so on their own. Many change to moderate, controlled use despite the assumption by professionals in the field that abstinence is the desirable if not the only outcome. There are, it seems, many influences on behaviour and change including those within the individual (e.g. motivation, creativity), within their lives (e.g. stress, opportunities), those around them (e.g. family, friends) and the context in which they live (e.g. treatment services, social policies). These various factors can encourage or deter change. The wise counsellor or psychotherapist views themselves as a humble catalyst to accelerate the natural process of an individual's personal growth and development in choosing wellbeing over harm.[3]

What are the main structured counselling approaches in substance misuse?

The four main approaches considered are as follow:

- motivational enhancement therapy
- solution focused therapy
- twelve step facilitation
- community reinforcement approach.

Motivational enhancement therapy (MET)

This approach aims to mobilise the individual's own resources to bring about the changes needed to achieve a non-user status. It assumes that the client has the necessary skills but needs encouragement to put them into practice. The task for the therapist is to provide a supportive, collaborative atmosphere in which the client's motivation can grow.

Motivational enhancement therapy is based on the work of William Miller[4,5] and Bien et al.[6] It combines the following three elements:

- stages of change
- motivational interviewing
- features of successful brief interventions.

These are discussed below.

Stages of change

Prochaska and DiClemente identified several stages in the behaviour change of people trying to stop smoking cigarettes.[7] These stages have been used in a wide range of behaviour change settings and are listed as follows.

- **Precontemplation**: Where the client does not think they have a problem despite some negative consequences of their behaviour. People at this stage often do not engage with services or attend because they are under some pressure to do so.

- **Contemplation**: Where the client has begun to recognise that there is a problem and that they need to consider change.
- **Preparation**: Where the client is beginning to try some changes. There may be some plans which are amended in the light of earlier successful or unsuccessful attempts.
- **Action**: Where the client acts on their plans.
- **Maintenance**: Where the client is sustaining change.
- **Relapse**: Where the client returns to the behaviour of the precontemplation stage. A lesser form of return to precontemplation is known as a 'lapse' or 'blip' which is a common occurrence in any behavioural change and is a temporary break in the plan. Most clients have at least one lapse and a wise practitioner will have 'inoculated' the client against a full relapse by establishing a relapse prevention plan.

The stages of change list is a useful guide to where the client might be in terms of change. Of course, this may not be a static position. Most dieters are in 'action' mode after a meal but may be 'Pre-contemplators' just before a meal is begun.

Motivational interviewing (MI)

This is an approach that directly addresses the ambivalence of change where people cannot understand why despite wanting to, they are 'unable' to change. It emphasises a non-directive, supportive reflective style for therapists. The tasks of the therapist are to:

- elicit the client's own statements about the problem(s)
- accentuate the discrepancy between the client's current and desired behaviours
- avoid or minimise confrontation
- 'roll' with resistance
- facilitate optimism and confidence in the client's own abilities.

Motivational interviewing also emphasises the importance of establishing the client's:

- readiness to change – is this change important?
- willingness to change – has the change started?
- ability to change – have they the confidence to persist?

The skills used include careful listening, affirming or acknowledging the client's views, asking open-ended questions (ones that do not elicit a 'yes' or 'no' answer) and developing 'talk' relating to change.

The avoidance of confrontation acknowledges Miller's findings that a client becomes more resistant or less open to change when a practitioner is arguing for change, being the 'expert', using shaming or blaming strategies, labelling the client or being in a hurry.

Features of successful brief interventions

These can be summarised by the acronym 'FRAMES' as follows.

F	feedback	assessment and information given to the client
R	responsibility	emphasising that the client has choices
A	advice	explicit advice on how to change behaviour
M	menu	offering alternative strategies
E	empathy	stance and support of the counsellor
S	self-efficacy	instilling optimism and hope

Solution focused therapy (SFT)

This therapy adopts the stance that the client is an 'expert' and can solve their problems with support. The approach involves looking for instances in the client's life where the problem does not occur or where solutions are in place. The therapist's task is to look for the client's resources and coping strategies and to help in identifying and supporting more use of these.

The underlying assumptions in SFT are that causation and history are not essential to successful outcomes. The more important issue is where the client is going; the possible and preferred futures. The client is not a 'problem' but a source of unique skills.

In SFT the therapist acknowledges the client's distress but talks more about:

- any instances when the distress is reduced
- exceptional circumstances – when the client feels well, calm or happy
- rating positive and negative experiences on scales to encourage a sense of perspective (e.g. 'How good are you feeling now on a scale of zero to ten, where zero is the worst you have ever felt and ten is the best you have ever felt?')
- the positive attributes the client is showing including courage, strength, honesty, resilience and persistence and complimenting the client for these.

The SFT strategies are chosen to help clients to think more positively about ways in which they can help themselves and to give them the confidence and hope to keep trying. Steve de Shazer and others developed this work in clinical practice when they realised that their clients were helped just as effectively by engaging in talk about the future (which could be changed) than in the past (which couldn't).[8] They realised that clients often avoid thinking about 'problems' because these are too upsetting. The approach includes the use of the 'miracle question':

> Imagine when you go to sleep one night a miracle happens and the problems we've been talking about disappear. As you were asleep, you did not know that a miracle had happened. When you woke up what would be the first signs for you that a miracle had happened?
>
> - What would you see?
> - How would things be different?
> - What would you do?

This is a useful way to achieve several of the aims of successful therapy in that it helps to clarify the desired goals and implies that these goals are achievable. Solution focused therapy can be used as a brief intervention when opportunities arise in any care context in which behavioural change is desirable.

Twelve step facilitation (TSF)

This intervention is based on the twelve step principle of Alcoholics Anonymous (AA) and is delivered as an individual psychotherapy provided by a trained therapist or counsellor. Alcoholics Anonymous is a group self-help programme available all over the world. For many people AA is the only support ever used to overcome a drinking problem and there is growing evidence of its effectiveness.

Twelve step facilitation has three main objectives based on the following first three steps.

- To facilitate '**acceptance**': This includes the realisation that alcohol has made life unmanageable, that will-power alone will not solve the problem and that abstinence is necessary.
- To facilitate '**surrender**': This includes giving oneself over to a higher power, accepting the fellowship offered by AA and following the twelve step programme.
- To instil '**hope**': This involves individuals examining their thinking patterns, emotions, behaviours, relationships, social activities and spirituality. These are examined to see how they relate to drinking and what changes are needed.

The task of the therapist is to guide the client to look at the following.

- Their family background and its influence.
- The enabling behaviours by others that support continued drinking.
- Changing routines and social contacts to remove alcohol as the main focus.
- Emotions that threaten change (e.g. HALT – hunger, anger, loneliness, tiredness).
- A moral inventory of the 'wrongs' done when drinking and resolving the resulting guilt that might threaten recovery.

The tasks given to the client will include diaries, assigned readings and written homework between sessions.

The community reinforcement approach (CRA)

This is a treatment approach that aims to help people achieve change by eliminating positive reinforcement or rewards for substance misuse and enhancing the rewards for alternatives. It integrates several treatment components including:

- motivation enhancement
- initiating change
- analysing drinking patterns
- increasing rewards
- learning new coping behaviours
- involving significant others (e.g. friends, family, partners, spouses).

Several studies have provided evidence for this approach. The community reinforcement approach has been used successfully together with a variety of other approaches including family therapy. This approach has been adopted widely in the USA and is beginning to be used in the UK.

What are the major types of formal psychological therapies?

The main four types discussed are:

- psychodynamic psychotherapy
- cognitive behavioural therapy
- cognitive analytic therapy
- systemic or family therapy.

Psychodynamic psychotherapy

Sigmund Freud conceptualised psychological distress as the result of conflicts within the person usually arising from their childhood. He set out a structural model of the mind as consisting of three parts.

- The **id**: A mainly unconscious energy reserve derived from instinctive drives whose aim is to maximise pleasure by satisfying these drives. The main drives relate to sex, death and the preservation of life.
- **The superego**: A mainly conscious moral energy reserve whose aim is to follow the rules laid down by parental and social restraints.
- **The ego**: This part of the mind is both conscious and unconscious and it has the aim of mediating between the demands of the id and superego to ensure preservation of the person in the world.

Freud also described the methods used by distressed people to try to cope with imbalances among these forces. The aim of therapy in Freud's model was the reconstruction of the client's personality using the therapeutic relationship and transference and countertransference experiences.

Transference is described as:

> an unconscious process in which the client transfers to the therapist feelings, emotions and attitudes that were experienced and/or desired in the client's childhood.

Countertransference is described as:

> the therapist's own feelings, emotions and attitudes to the patient.

The therapist's task was to analyse the client to identify the unresolved conflicts and help the client towards resolution.

Psychodynamic psychotherapy has developed to become more focused these days on helping clients to understand conflicts in their feelings, desires and beliefs and how these affect their relationships with others. The interaction between the therapist and client provides a basis for greater self-awareness.

Cognitive behavioural therapy (CBT)

This form of therapy focuses on the links between physical reactions, feelings, thoughts and behaviour that are formed by learning and which are maintained by the consequences of behaviour. Thoughts or cognitions are seen as central to the functioning of individuals. Problems arise from the meanings that individuals give to events not the events themselves. These meanings are derived from the framework of core beliefs and assumptions that have been developed during the individual's childhood and adult years. The therapy developed from the work of Aaron Beck and there are now many cognitive therapies arising from his work. A wide range of problems and disorders has been treated using CBT and there is a substantial evidence base to support its use in many areas of health practice.

Central to the application of CBT is the case formulation which reflects the therapist's hypothesis about the client's difficulties. It is assumed that during early development underlying assumptions and core beliefs develop which make the individual vulnerable to certain negative life events. The negative life event is then a trigger which causes 'negative automatic thoughts' to be activated. These give rise to unhelpful ways of feeling and behaving.

The task of the therapist in CBT is to help the client identify the unhelpful cognitions and to develop new, positive cognitions that give rise to more positive experiences of the self, others and the world.

A range of cognitive and behavioural strategies include the following.

- **Guided discovery**: Where the therapist asks questions to challenge the client's thinking.
- **Behavioural experiments**: Where clients 'try out' a new behaviour, or agree to behave in a way that challenges their beliefs (for example, the therapist accompanying an agoraphobic client to a supermarket and remaining there together until the client's panic subsides and he or she understands that they can manage their emotions effectively).
- **Self monitoring**: Diaries are kept by the client to encourage objectivity, perspective and learning.
- **Activity scheduling**: Clients plan activities to counter 'safety behaviours', or avoidance of life and the world.

Cognitive analytic therapy (CAT)

This therapy brings together psychodynamic and cognitive approaches in a systematic way. It uses psychodynamic concepts to examine repetitive cycles of behaviour which perpetuate negative or unhelpful ways of thinking and behaving. The therapy evolved from the work of Antony Ryle.[9]

In CAT the internalised learning that a person develops during childhood is known as reciprocal role procedures (RRP). These RRPs are based on the caregiving relationships that the client experienced as a child. Affectionate care will lead to a positive expectation about self and others ('My Mum/Dad loves me' leads to 'I'm a loveable person and I know how to love others'), whereas other forms of care might produce a different response ('My Mum/Dad hates me' might lead to 'I'm not loveable, so nobody could love me'). These underlying, possibly unconscious beliefs can influence behaviour in subtle ways. The therapist's task is to detect the underlying and observable aspects of the client's life, help make sense of them and encourage change.

Three main stages are involved in CAT.

- **Reformulation**: This involves a careful examination of the issues in the client's life and sharing these with the client.
- **Recognition**: This involves looking at the themes and patterns in the client's life using diaries. The therapist helps the client to notice the roles they adopt and any 'dilemmas, traps and snags' that regularly occur. Dilemmas, traps and snags are three common self-damaging ways of relating to oneself and others.
- **Revision**: This involves the encouragement and practising of new ways of thinking, feeling and behaving.

The therapist supports the client in practising the changes and therapy ends with a 'goodbye letter' to summarise the learning.

Systemic or family therapy (ST)

This approach involves focusing on the connections between people and relationships in the different contexts that occur such as couples, families, schools, care settings and wider systems. The approach looks at how changes in one part of a 'system' or set of relationships produce changes elsewhere, sometimes predictably and positively, at other times unexpectedly and negatively. Systemic therapy is used with couples and families in a range of ways including where there are childhood problems, in substance misuse and where a family is in conflict and struggling to cope. Each individual family member contributes to the overall family system and 'the whole is greater than the sum of its parts'.

The task of the therapist is to look for:

- **Relationship patterns**: In terms of where in the family system people are close and where they are not.
- **Belief systems**: In terms of the family's view of the world or their 'script', their traditions, myths and shared assumptions and how these regulate family activity.
- **Context**: In terms of the meaning, to the family, of the distress being experienced. Context is examined in terms of culture (e.g. ethnicity and faith), the family script, the individual scripts of family members, the relationships between them, the life events they have and are encountering, the repeating patterns in the family's life and the behaviours they engage in.

Systemic therapy sees distress as having a homeostatic function preventing changes in a family around the time of major life events. Transitions are a part of family life and may be common (e.g. the birth of a child or an older child leaving home). Most families cope with these readjustments after a period of some uncertainty. However, some transitions may be harder to adjust to (e.g. redundancy, chronic illness or death).

The therapist's task is to provide insight, clarify the situation and its meaning and to suggest or prescribe tasks that aim to help the family use its own strengths to solve its problems. The approach acknowledges that both the family and the therapist have expertise that can be usefully combined.

The therapy aims to identify patterns in family relationships and behaviour. It accepts that every member may have a different view, that all views are valid and offers a different perspective, which empowers the family to make changes.

What evidence is there for the efficacy of talking treatments?

There have been several reviews summarising the evidence for the efficacy of talking treatments both in general and in substance misuse more specifically.

The general reviews can be found elsewhere.[10,11] In substance misuse an early indication of the usefulness of talking treatments came in 1996 in the *Effectiveness Review* which identified benefits from 'cognitive behavioural approaches, twelve step addiction counselling, Gesalt and family therapy'.[12] More recent reviews commissioned by the NTA have summarised research findings, mainly from the USA to help inform service providers.[13,14]

In relation to methadone the findings suggest that there are several elements of successful treatment:

> Most opioid users seeking treatment present to services with a range of problems including severe family and social problems, employment difficulties and use of other illicit drugs. Many have co-morbid psychiatric disorders, or other co-morbidity (e.g. HIV or hepatitis C infection). These problems may impede the progress of service users and work against their retention in treatment. Retention is acknowledged as having a major association with good outcomes.[13]

It has been found that the more successful methadone treatments are those that reflect a good organisational management, through providing a range of services that maximise the effectiveness of methadone and can improve client outcomes. These include counselling and other psychosocial interventions and provision of 'ancillary' services.[13]

Cocaine/crack dependence also benefits from talking treatments:[14]

> Drug-free psychosocial interventions such as counselling, provided on a non-residential basis, are the most cost-effective options for clients with few complicating problems.

There are also findings that suggest that all staff involved with clients who misuse substances can contribute to the overall effectiveness of any service with the right attitude and approach with even brief client contact.

> Most of the research into the effectiveness of opportunistic brief interventions (OBIs) has been with general populations in a wide range of settings and countries, but a recent study at a needle exchange provided the first direct evidence that brief interventions can produce decreases in alcohol use among active injecting drug users with drinking problems.[15]

> Opportunistic interventions can usefully include a more person-centred, motivational component to begin the process of the client considering whether or not to change. Rollnick *et al.* have adapted key features of motivational interviewing to be applicable to brief health promotion interventions.[16] Such an approach is more likely to fit well with the

non-judgemental, enabling culture of many community drug agencies, than an authoritative, advice-based approach.[17]

Engagement of clients in treatment has been shown to be strongly influenced by the approach adopted by service staff.

Rapid intake to treatment, motivational interventions, active intensive on-going support, as well as practical measures to encourage attendance are all approaches that research suggests can impact positively on engagement. Factors such as empathic, positive staff approaches and flexible, responsive services have been associated with more positive outcomes for clients. The attitudes of the staff and keyworkers can also influence engagement of drug users in services positively. Poor response to treatment can be a legitimate response to poor treatment. Much depends on the therapy and the setting. But much also depends on whether treatment is delivered quickly after presentation, and with understanding and optimism.

This research summary suggests that practitioners and services have a wide range of responses available to minimise poor engagement and retention. The research suggests that low retention figures should appropriately lead to a review of the attitudes and characteristics of the service among other factors. The simple assumption that such problems are only due to poorly motivated drug users is difficult to sustain.[17]

The NTA research findings on treating cocaine/crack dependence also emphasise the importance of an empathic approach and availability of structured counselling.[14]

Although there is no magic bullet, cocaine misuse is treatable. Rather than nothing working, it is more that any approaches already familiar to drug services in Britain work well but none are specific to the treatment of crack dependence.

- There is little understanding of how to prompt initial contact with treatment services, but once contact is made, rapid intake, proactive reminders, and practical help with attendance have improved treatment uptake rates.
- Once they start treatment, clients tend to stay longer and respond better if they feel that their keyworker is empathic and understanding, underlying the crucial role workers play in motivating and retaining clients.

Opportunistic brief interventions (OBIs)

Opportunistic brief interventions:

take place outside specialist alcohol agencies and are directed at people who have not sought help for their alcohol use. They may take only a few minutes, but can be longer. Typically, they include an enquiry into the client's drinking, giving information and feedback relating to their consumption and risk level, and finally, advice on how to reduce risks.[18]

The evidence for the effectiveness of treatment for alcohol misuse is now well established. What is now interesting researchers is the best 'fit' of client needs, therapists, and therapeutic approaches. An impressive ten-year long study in the USA, Project Match, looked at the outcomes from 1726 clients undergoing post-detox. therapy with 81 Masters level therapists using one of three approaches; motivational enhancement therapy, cognitive behavioural therapy or twelve step facilitation. Two years after the therapeutic treatments each had achieved similar levels of success.[18] Motivational enhancement has also been studied extensively with good outcomes.[5]

The role of the practice counsellor

It is clear that structured counselling is now seen as an essential element of substance misuse services and other services where behaviour change is desirable within primary care. In this there is an important role for the practice counsellor.

Depending on the skills and training of the practice counsellor there are a variety of roles that they might adopt:

* helping individual clients
* helping couples
* helping families
* running groups
* providing advice to clients and others on the telephone
* advising other staff in the practice about their own clients
* producing written information for clients
* producing written information for staff
* advising the practice on becoming or remaining psychologically aware
* training others.

The practice counsellor needs to ask themselves the following questions.

* What are the needs of the clients in this practice?
* What are the needs of the staff?
* What does the practice need?
* Which of these needs can I meet?
* How shall I prioritise my time?
* How can I maintain my effectiveness?

Obviously these questions cannot be answered by the practice counsellor alone and require input from staff, managers and clinicians. The amount of time available will also be an issue as will the knowledge, expectations and psychological sophistication of all concerned. It is usually the case that a confident professional is able to listen to advice from others and make their own decision about whether or not to take it.

Practice counsellors have to consider their own needs. They may have to be diplomatic and cautious about their role. They can often be 'lone practitioners'. It is important that they are supported both managerially and by clinical supervision. This supervision may take several forms including one to one sessions with a senior, experienced colleague or in a group of peers. The supervision is a vital part of learning and renewal to ensure that the practice counsellor is able to give their clients a good service without feeling 'drained' or 'burnt out'.

In whichever way the practice counsellor decides to proceed, whoever they work with (clients, staff or the practice as an organisation), and whichever therapeutic model they use there will be a series of stages common to the work. These stages have been identified by Velleman as follows:[19]

- developing trust
- exploring problem areas
- helping to set goals
- empowering into action
- helping to maintain change
- agreeing when to end.

Developing trust is the most important stage as without trust the client won't or can't talk about their worries and fears. Trust is encouraged by looking at people, listening carefully, showing respect, allowing silences and by summarising what we have heard from the client. If this is done with warmth, understanding and genuineness the client is invited to overcome their reticence and accept help. After this the specific approaches to use can evolve from the needs of the client and the skills, knowledge and experience of the client and practice counsellor.

A toolkit for primary care staff involved in substance misuse

It is clear that there are ways in which all staff in primary care can help to contribute to an effective service. A toolkit of approaches would include:

- a positive, respectful attitude
- an assumption that the individual will change one day and the communication of hope
- bearing in mind that ambivalence is natural
- helping individuals to work out their own cost-benefit analysis to look at:
  - the positives of change
  - the negatives of change
  - the positives of staying the same
  - the negatives of staying the same
  (If the change was all positive and staying the same was all negative, there would be no ambivalence. The important things to identify are the positives of staying the same (as 'good' things will be lost by changing) and the negatives of change (as these are barriers to change)
- bearing in mind the stages of change and using strategies appropriately:
  - pre-contemplation: ask why other people think there is a problem
  - contemplation: ask about the cost-benefit analysis
  - decision making: ask what practical changes could be made
  - action: ask about any successes however small
  - maintenance: ask about how a lapse would be handled to prevent relapse

- remember to notice any positives
  - you're looking well
  - you're on time today
- asking rather than telling – when people give answers they are clarifying their own thinking
- remember 'FRAMES':
  - F   feedback
  - R   responsibility
  - A   advice
  - M   menu
  - E   empathy
  - S   self-efficacy.

Using these tools can help to ensure that all client contacts contribute to a supportive approach.

References

1   Department of Health (2004) *Organising and Delivering Psychological Therapies.* Department of Health, London.
2   Department of Health (2002) *Models of Care.* DoH, London.
3   Heather N and Stockwell T (eds) (2004) *The Essential Handbook of Treatment and Prevention of Alcohol Problems.* John Wiley and Sons, Chichester.
4   Miller WR (1985) Motivation for treatment: a review with special emphasis on alcoholism. *Psychological Bulletin.* **98**: 85–107.
5   Miller WR and Rollnick S (2002) *Motivational Interviewing* (2e). The Guilford Press, New York.
6   Bien TH, Miller WR and Tonigan JS (1993) Brief interventions for alcohol problems: a review. *Addiction.* **88**: 315–36.
7   Prochaska J and DiClemente C (1986) Towards a comprehensive model of change. In: WR Miller and N Heather (eds) *Treating Addictive Behaviours: processes of change.* Plenum, New York.
8   de Shazer S (1985) *Keys to Solutions in Brief Therapy.* WW Norton, New York.
9   Ryle A (1990) *Cognitive Analytic Therapy: active participation in change.* John Wiley and Sons, Chichester.
10 Roth A and Fonagy P (1996) *What Works for Whom? A Critical Review of Psychotherapy Research.* The Guilford Press, New York.
11 Department of Health (2001) *Treatment Choice in Psychological Therapies and Counselling: evidence based clinical practice guideline.* Department of Health, London.
12 *Effectiveness Review* (1996).
13 National Treatment Agency (2002) *More Than Just Methadone Dose: enhancing outcomes of methadone maintenance treatment with counselling and 'ancillary' services.* National Treatment Agency, London.
14 National Treatment Agency (2004) *Treating cocaine/crack dependence. Research in Practice No. 1a.* Drug Services' Briefing. National Treatment Agency, London.

15 Stein MD, Charuvastra A, Maksad J *et al.* (2002) A randomised trial of a brief alcohol intervention for needle exchanges (BRAINE). *Addiction.* **97**(6): 691–700.

16 Rollnick S, Mason P and Butler C (1999) *Health Behaviour Change: a guide for practitioners.* Churchill Livingstone, London.

17 National Treatment Agency (2004) *Engaging and Retaining Clients in Drug Treatment.* National Treatment Agency, London.

18 Babor TF and Del Boca FK (2003) *Treatment Matching in Alcoholism.* Cambridge University Press, Cambridge.

19 Velleman R (2001) *Counselling for Alcohol Problems.* Sage, London.

CHAPTER 10

Special issues for effective treatment of homeless drug users

Angela Jones

Introduction

There is a terrible logic which links substance misuse, in its broadest sense, with homelessness. All the available data confirm a higher prevalence of one with the other than in the general population, although opinions vary as to which is the chicken and which is the egg. What is certain is that homeless people with substance misuse problems rank among the most socially excluded in our society and present a huge challenge to those trying to provide them with the healthcare they so desperately need.

The challenge

There is no doubt that homeless people have higher rates of many health problems than the population as a whole. During the late 1980s and early 1990s numerous UK studies established this, culminating in the 1994 report of the Royal College of Physicians Working Party, *Homelessness and Ill Health*.[1]

Despite their acknowledged massive load of morbidity, homeless people are prone to be victims of the 'Inverse Care Law' described by Tudor Hart in his seminal work on health and social exclusion.[2] This law states that health care is available in inverse proportion to the healthcare needs of a population. In the case of homeless people the lack of access to healthcare revolves around a number of factors.

- Doctors' attitudes towards treating homeless people: a study in Avon in 1997 showed that GPs perceive homeless patients to be challenging in terms of social problems (90% of respondents agreed), the lack of medical records (88% agreed), the complex health problems (79% agreed) and the associated alcohol or substance misuse (78% agreed).[3] Lester has looked at this using qualitative techniques and concluded that GPs' attitudes and consultation behaviour toward the homeless were a major barrier to achieving good healthcare, possibly more important than the attitudes of reception staff and the perceived inadequacies of 'the system'.[4]
- Homeless people are often circumspect in seeking healthcare. This can be because of other priorities, or because of past bad experiences when attempting to access medical services.

- Healthcare provision has, in the past, militated against homeless people accessing good healthcare. In particular the remuneration structure for GPs acted as a disincentive to registering homeless patients.[3] This has been addressed more recently by new contracting arrangements for primary care (*see* below). Also, hospital services find it difficult to manage homeless patients due to difficulties with on-going care arrangements because of the lack of accommodation.

Thus, we have a population of people with huge healthcare needs who either cannot or will not access the means to address them. By looking at the provision of care for substance misuse problems and homeless people, it is possible to review the various models that can be used to address the problems.

Models of treatment services

Substance misuse is inextricably linked into the homelessness story of many of the individuals who find themselves homeless in the UK. The fact is that, just as simply putting a homeless person into accommodation does not amount to their reintegration into society, the provision of instant across-the-board detoxification or substitute prescribing for every homeless drug user would not alone be the solution to their problems. There are no 'quick fixes' for this situation. In fact, a chaotic injecting heroin user is arguably safer using in the street or a night shelter, where an ambulance will be called if he overdoses, than in the kind of lonely bedsit or 'bed and breakfast' accommodation which is the mainstay of emergency temporary accommodation.

An individual who has undergone the sort of prolonged social degradation that leads to them sleeping rough and dependent on heroin and crack on our streets will generally need long term engagement with robust holistic services which can provide seamless care for their social, psychological, psychiatric and physical needs. Ideally, these agencies would also see the spiritual wellbeing of the client as important and would act as a focus for their reintegration into society. Although this is clearly a tall order, I would contend that it is achievable. However, the model applied, be it a 'one-stop-shop' or an integrated care pathway between different agencies in any particular locality, will depend on local factors. What is important is that such services are actively planned and appropriately resourced, and that the staff working in them are very well supported.

In the one-stop-shop model, the homeless person is able to access their physical, psychological, social and spiritual needs through a single agency. This agency would ideally be situated within a primary care setting, given that, in the UK NHS, the GP is probably the last of the medical generalists and remains the 'gatekeeper' to secondary care for his/her patients.

Furthermore, primary care is a direct access service, allowing homeless people to access help at the point of need, with a minimum of bureaucracy or delay. A GP working alone could not provide the level of service required. Such services can only be offered in a sustainable fashion by a well-developed and highly-skilled multi-disciplinary primary healthcare team.

The personal medical services (PMS) model of primary care provision, piloted in the late 1990s and now established permanently as a model of provision, has allowed for considerable flexibility and innovation in provision for disadvantaged patient groups, leading to the establishment of significant numbers of specialist primary care services for homeless people across the UK.[5] The ideal of medical, psychiatric, dental, podiatric and welfare provision available at one venue has been aspired to and met in varying extents by various innovative organisations, limited as they are by local pressures. Most will aim to ensure effective linkage to the services they cannot provide themselves on site and should offer advocacy, particularly when relating to statutory agencies such as housing or benefits agencies.

Within this kind of primary care provision, staff will request and record information regarding the past and current medical history, including any substance misuse problems. This gives an opportunity for brief interventions including harm reduction advice relating to the stated issues. Many patients will not be seeking treatment for their substance misuse but can be reassured that treatment will be forthcoming should their attitude change in the future. If the patient is already clear that they are interested in formal treatment for a substance misuse problem, they can then be referred for assessment via whatever care pathway is in place for that organisation. These are likely to become more streamlined under the new system of *Models of Care* currently being developed and implemented by the NTA.

The way in which practices provide services for substance misuse currently varies, depending on the local pattern of provision. The two main models are similar to those in mainstream primary care: referral to a specialist agency or treatment within the primary care setting. Treatment by a specialist agency has the advantage of consultant-led care and easy access to help for co-morbid mental health problems. However, secondary care agencies may not have expertise in care of homeless people, will be less effective at harm reduction and health promotion activities and may well lack the flexibility necessary to engage this highly chaotic group. In-house primary care provision is described in Chapter 2. It has the obvious advantage of dovetailing into primary care services but may not be suitable for certain patients. Which patients are deemed unsuitable will depend on the facilities, expertise and local circumstances of the service but may include injectable opiate prescribing, benzodiazepine maintenance and complex co-morbid conditions, including severe personality disorder. Finally, various hybrid patterns have arisen, dictated by local circumstances, most typically unacceptably long waiting times for specialist assessment. It is likely that these will gradually become regularised with improved funding of treatment and strenuous efforts at standardisation of treatment by the NTA. However, hopefully there will still be room for innovation in response to local need.

Substance misuse and the homeless: the patient journey

It can be helpful to think about three phases when managing a homeless person with addiction problems:

- engagement
- retention
- mainstreaming.

Stage 1: engagement

The first phase is that of engaging the homeless substance misuser in treatment. This can take considerable time, given that the motivation may not be high in a homeless person who has many other priorities in life such as finding food, funds and shelter and avoiding persons or situations which pose a risk to their safety. The primary care setting has an advantage in this engagement phase, as the patient will often need to approach their local medical centre for acute care for complications of their homelessness or substance misuse, or for help with obtaining certification related to fitness for work. Few homeless substance misusers would realistically be capable of work and thus approach GPs for a 'Med 3' (sick note or paper) to state that they are not fit for work. This gives the GP an opportunity to monitor the person's health closely by giving relatively short Med 3s of four weeks' (or less) duration. Each subsequent review interview is then an opportunity to discuss harm minimisation and treatment options, in the hope of gradually obtaining the patient's trust and advancing the process of engagement.

As is clear from the above, the process of engagement starts at registration with a primary care provider. It is essential that the practice has well-developed mechanisms for obtaining information regarding the patient from their previous primary care team. This process will of course require explicit signed consent from the patient. The process can be streamlined by training team members to conduct the initial registration interview, which is also an opportunity to demonstrate the holistic and non-judgemental stance of the practice, and also to give important information about the practice such as opening times, how to obtain appointments, repeat prescriptions and Med 3s, etc.

However, significant numbers of homeless people are engaged initially in treatment by the numerous non-statutory agencies set up to deliver help, services and advice to both homeless and housed substance misusers. Providers of temporary housing (shelters and hostels) have made strenuous efforts to ensure that their staff have training in addiction related issues and will often enable service users to make contact with relevant agencies. The pathways by which a homeless person will obtain treatment will vary according to local provision, but as mentioned previously, should become more streamlined under *Models of Care*.

What kind of service will encourage a homeless person to use it? Experience stresses the importance of a warm and welcoming ambience and a non-judgemental attitude among the workers. Frontline staff, such as receptionists, are key in transmitting this to the patients and these staff need special attention in terms of training, support and affirmation. Clinicians need to be prepared to be patient-led in terms of interventions, but need to be supported by clear practice guidelines in terms of what can and cannot be prescribed, and when, in order to maintain safe practice in the face of potentially challenging scenarios. Finally, procedures need to be flexible in order to be able to provide care when the patient is willing to accept it. Opportunistic interventions are far more likely to happen than those arranged by appointment.

Once a substance misuser has decided to ask for treatment, the question arises as to how soon a full assessment should be offered (*see* Chapter 2 for more information). Little evidence is available on this question. What seems to be clear is that to prescribe substitute opiates without a proper assessment is to lay oneself and the patient open to a host of dangers. The only exception to the 'no-assessment, no prescription' rule would be the scenario where a patient arrives on a current prescription from elsewhere, which is verifiable. These circumstances are more likely to occur in a homeless or travelling person, with their increased mobility and necessity to move due to risk to personal safety or economic factors. Verifying such prescriptions may require a considerable input of staff time and is one of the factors which needs to be considered when setting up such a service.

Stage 2: retention

With research indicating successful outcomes being related to retention in treatment, it is clear that it is very important to maximise retention in treatment as far as is possible.[6] What factors lead to retention in the homeless patient group? Evidence specific to homeless patients is limited.[7] The same factors which promote engagement would seem logically to be related also to retention. However, the quality of the relationship between the patient and their keyworker is even more relevant. This worker will have regular meetings with the patient and will have the opportunity not only to engage about the current issues but also to build up a relationship of trust which enables the patient, at their own pace, to look at past issues and life events. They will be able to help the patient to stabilise their lifestyle, minimise harms, seek accommodation, undertake more enhancing daily activities and ultimately to obtain gainful employment. They can also prompt the patient to seek urgent or routine medical review, as required. This is clearly a tall order for a single individual and supportive management as well as being part of a flexible multi-disciplinary team is vital to maximise the benefits of treatment to the patient. In particular, easy access to medical, nursing and social care is necessary. Care planning, with regular review involving the patient, is key to managing this complex scenario and thus in promoting retention. Similarly, excellent communication between team members, enabled by the use of IT, is essential.

What about prescribing? Is it necessary to prescribe what the patient demands in order to retain them in treatment? The answer to this is that each agency needs to have clear and transparent guidelines or protocols on what it is prepared to prescribe. Team members need to keep to these guidelines as far as is possible. The community of substance misusers is a closeknit one – and none more so than that of homeless substance misusers. If word reaches the street that a certain doctor is willing to prescribe hard-to-obtain medication, that doctor will soon have many more requests. Likewise, it is demoralising for teams which are trying to maintain their boundaries to be let down by a team member's lax decision. On the other hand, exceptions do occasionally occur and teams need to listen to their colleagues if a justifiable variation from the usual policy seems to be indicated.

It can be helpful to defuse this kind of difficult consultation if practice guidelines state that a team discussion will be held if a prescription request is outside the guidelines. The clinician must then, of course, be willing to abide by the decision of the team. Our experience is that it is rare to lose a patient from treatment due to refusal to prescribe, as long as they are given an explanation of the reasons for refusal and there is an opportunity for discussing an alternative strategy for dealing with the problem. The maintenance of strict guidelines can involve some tough interactions for doctors and nurses with patients but these are ultimately far less draining than the continual round of bargaining and confrontation that accompanies a more relaxed policy.

Stage 3: mainstreaming

When does a homeless patient with substance misuse cease to be a special patient needing special input from a bespoke agency? Some may argue that once a homeless person has been housed, their needs return to those of an 'ordinary' person. This does not seem to be the case in practice, firstly, because the person takes into their accommodated situation the same difficulties, whether social, psychological or physical, that took them into homelessness in the first place, and secondly, because being accommodated is not necessarily 'normative' for a homeless person. They may not have the skills of self-sufficiency, money management, self-care or personal boundary-setting that are required to maintain a tenancy, and will need special input and monitoring to ensure that they do not experience the well known revolving door straight back into homelessness. These transitions generally require the involvement of non-statutory agencies who, depending on local resources, can provide support, although usually on a time-limited basis.

Furthermore, although all patient-clinician relationships are special, it follows that the transition from socially excluded homeless substance misuser to housed member of society is such a fundamental one that the relationship with the therapist or therapeutic organisation which supported you in this phase is extremely strong and not easily broken. Our experience is that patients can break their ties with their homeless provider once they have to, because of geographical factors, or when they find that to attend the premises becomes too challenging (particularly in terms of triggers and other service users). It is rarely advisable to force the issue of 'moving on' unless one of these factors comes into play; the patient will ultimately move on when they are ready.

Special issues
Alcohol

Alcohol is an important factor in the addiction picture for many homeless patients. It is a fact of life in the homeless environment, with many homeless people having primary alcohol problems. Even if the patient is not using alcohol at the time of assessment, it is extremely common, if not the norm, for alcohol use to creep in as substitute prescribing is instituted and street drug usage decreases. This may be 'straightforward' cross-addiction or may represent the patient needing another psychotropic substance to address an underlying and emerging mental health problem. This is borne out by data from the NTORS study.[8] Alcohol use adds to the risk of opiate substitute prescribing and is strongly to be avoided in chronic hepatitis C infection. It needs to be carefully managed and the use of an alcohol breathalyser can be an excellent tool to monitor alcohol intake both during negotiation regarding prescriptions and for managing community alcohol detoxification.

Medicines management

Homeless people live in a dangerous and threatening environment. Carrying medication is accompanied by the risk of losing it, having it stolen, or being tempted to sell it in order to raise money (diversion). Any prescribing for homeless people needs to take these factors into account.

- The first rule is that 'lost' medicines of any kind should not automatically be replaced. Claims of stolen medicines need to be supported by a police report. A pattern of having 'divertable' medicines repeatedly lost or stolen should lead to a review of prescribing and possible suspension of the prescription.
- Secondly, medication should be prescribed, wherever possible, to a place of safety. Many hostels and shelters will, after discussion with the clinician, hold medications for their residents. Concordance is greatly enhanced by provision of medication in blister packs but this has financial implications for pharmacies and/or PCTs.
- Thirdly, where a place of safety is not available, daily scripts should be considered. Although time consuming, they have the advantage of minimising the risks (although hoarding with a view to overdose or diversion is still possible, unless consumption is supervised).
- Wherever possible, opiates should only be prescribed for supervised daily consumption. Even a take-away dose for Sunday causes significant difficulties for patients, with the risk of 'taxing' – people waiting outside pharmacies to steal, or buy, the take-away dose.
- Finally, given the uncertain world in which homeless people live and the complexity of their health needs, it is generally advisable to prescribe for short periods only. The period should depend chiefly on the length of time needed before the next review, which in turn may depend on the patient's social, psychological or physical state but will usually be between one day and two weeks, but rarely as long as a month.

Prevention and screening

Like other substance misusers, homeless people are at risk of contracting blood-borne virus infections such as hepatitis B, C and HIV. Hepatitis A can be a problem especially given the institutional nature of much of the available temporary accommodation. Hence, immunisation against hepatitis A and B are an integral part of the management of homeless substance misusers. The immunisation protocol used will depend on local patient group directions. There is some evidence that using an accelerated schedule enhances uptake.[9] Recently there has been a move among some specialist units to using combined hep. A/hep. B vaccines (*see* Chapter 4, page 51).

The advisability of screening for HIV and hepatitis C infections is less clear. Although this patient group is clearly at risk in view of both its risk of injecting drug use with shared equipment and also sexual transmission relating to sex work, some specialist agencies feel that blanket screening is not appropriate. The rationale for this is that informed consent involves making a decision that the patient is able to cope with the implications of a potential positive result. This cannot be assumed for homeless people who are living under extremely stressful conditions. Furthermore, many homeless people are not ready for or suitable for treatments currently available (particularly in the case of hepatitis C). Thus, a policy of testing on a case-by-case basis would seem to be most appropriate.

Catch-up for missed childhood immunisations can be an issue for younger homeless people, who are quite likely to have missed immunisations due to parental issues or truancy from school. Local recommendations should be sought from the local public health resources. Obtaining accurate information about immunisation history may be a challenge. In general, it is worthwhile to check young women for rubella antibodies with a view to immunisation if negative. Advice to use contraception and take folic acid supplementation if sexually active, should also be given (*see* Chapter 4 for information on harm reduction).

Chronic disease management

Substance misusers who are homeless are prone to chronic illnesses such as epilepsy, asthma or chronic obstructive pulmonary disease or chronic hepatitis C. Such health matters may easily be overlooked in the busy life of a substance misuser and it requires determination, organisation and sometimes an element of (gentle) persuasion to ensure that they are appropriately managed. Given that these patients probably attend the surgery every one or two weeks, it should be possible to ensure that a GP or practice nurse can see them to review their management, when necessary. It is usually most conducive to arrange medical appointments on the same day as the addiction appointment, to minimise the risk of non-attendance.

Psychiatric care

With diagnosed mental illness at an incidence of up to 50% in the homeless population, the incidence of co-morbidity between substance misuse and psychiatric illness is bound to be very high, particularly as many patients with significant mental illnesses remain undiagnosed while homeless due to their relative invisibility among the homeless population and their tendency to move around the country. Others may attract a diagnosis but this fails to be recorded anywhere which can be traced by services in another area. Traceability of records is further impeded by the lack of a national medical database and by the inconsistent use of names or dates of birth by the patient. However, with some detective work by an experienced and determined administrative worker, these difficulties are surprisingly often overcome.

When it comes to managing a homeless person who misuses drugs or alcohol and is exhibiting or experiencing psychiatric symptoms great levels of skills are required. These skills are often to be found in the specialist multi-disciplinary primary care teams who work with this group. However, these teams need easily-accessible expert help. This can take various forms:

- attached community psychiatric nurse working within the primary care team
- in-reach to the primary care team by psychiatric team, e.g. consultant clinics at the practice
- care planning meetings between the community mental health team and the practice team
- direct employment of a mental health specialist (usually RMN with community experience) within the practice team.

A combination of these models is often required to maintain adequate and safe management of these complex cases. What is universally vital is a mutual understanding and respect of both teams for each others' expertise – the psychiatrist is the expert in mental health but the homelessness team will be the experts in homelessness and often in the management of addiction in this group. Overall management decisions will need to pay due heed to both aspects of the patient's predicament. In addition, when a substance misuse issue is also present, a tripartite discussion also involving the team's addiction specialist will be necessary.

Rehabilitation services

When taking all the factors impinging on a homeless substance misuser into account, it would seem logical that a period of rehabilitation would be indicated in order to successfully complete their treatment. On the other hand, it is these very same factors that make appropriate referrals to rehabilitation for this group such a difficult issue. There are very few rehabilitation centres in the UK that will take 'dual diagnosis' clients – many homeless people fall into this category. Still fewer take pets (specifically dogs), which can act as a significant barrier to acceptance for homeless clients. Furthermore, the transition from the chaos of street homeless substance misuse to the highly structured environment of a rehabilitation centre may simply be too much to contemplate. Finally, abstinence may not be a realistic goal if the addiction treatment is at a relatively early stage.

For this reason a few pioneering 'pre-rehab.' providers have been developed. An example is the Drug Recovery Project in Oxford, a joint venture between a local direct-access housing provider and the local specialist primary healthcare provider for homeless people which aims to provide a slow detoxification from drugs of addiction in a supportive and structured abstinent residential setting. Key to the success of such projects is selection of clients for whom abstinence is a safe and preferred option to long-term methadone maintenance.

Prison

Many homeless people end up in prison and many prisoners are released to homelessness. Thus, relationships with the prison service, in particular the prison medical services, are vital for good through care. With the responsibility for prison healthcare falling to PCTs, this communication is becoming more of an achievable reality. There are still issues to be faced however, in particular the management of substance misusers in prison. Anecdotally, the policy of detoxification from methadone maintenance is still the rule in prisoners serving more than a very short term. This means that prisoners are often released to homelessness in an opiate naïve state, and, despite the delivery of education regarding overdose risk, this can result in opiate overdose soon after release and, all too often, in death.

Asylum seekers

The decision as to whether to treat asylum seekers and 'mainstream' homeless people in the same venue depends on local factors. There are significant drawbacks, however, in mixing the two populations. In particular, the environment within agencies managing homeless people can be challenging at times, and however well organised the agency, aggressive incidents do occur. This is clearly a very unsuitable scenario for asylum seekers, who will often be fleeing precisely this kind of environment. Distress and an unwillingness to attend the agency may well result. However, for asylum seekers who, for reasons of mental disorder, substance misuse or other factors, fail within their housing provision and become homeless, it may become most appropriate to manage them alongside mainstream homeless people, whilst taking into account, as far as possible, their individual problems and sensitivities.

Summary

Another terrible logic, to match the one with which this chapter began, is one which I have christened the 'Inverse Complexity Law'. This is a syndrome which has been observed anecdotally by many primary care practitioners working in the field of addiction and which mirrors Tudor Hart's Inverse Care Law. The Inverse Complexity Law states that the likelihood of a patient actually attending a specialist clinic is inversely proportional to the complexity of his or her case; in other words, primary care ends up treating very complex patients because it is the only place where these patients actually manage to attend! This highlights the need for a close working relationship between primary and secondary care providers, enabling the primary care workers in the field to feel supported and easily able to access help and advice when required. It also highlights the need for robust, flexible, well funded and appropriately supported primary care agencies, who will be ready and able to treat the homeless addict when they are ready and able to engage.

References

1   Royal College of Physicians (1994) *Homelessness and Ill Health*. Royal College of Physicians, London.
2   Tudor Hart J (1971) The Inverse Care Law. *Lancet*. **1**: 405–12.
3   Wood N, Wilkinson C and Kumar A (1997) Do the homeless get a fair deal from general practitioners? *J Roy Soc Health*. **117**: 292–7.
4   Lester H and Bradley C (2001) Barriers to primary healthcare for the homeless: the general practitioner's perspective. *Eur J Gen Prac*. **7**: 6–12.
5   Lester H, Wright N and Heath I (2002) Developments in the provision of primary health care for homeless people (editorial). *Br J Gen Pract*. **52**: 91–2.
6   Gossop M, Marsden J, Stewart D *et al.* (1999) Methadone treatment practices and outcome for opiate addicts treated in drug clinics and in general practice: results from the National Treatment Outcome Research Study. *Br J Gen Prac*. **49**: 31–4.
7   Neale J and Kennedy C (2002) Good practice towards homeless drug users: research evidence from Scotland. *Health and Social Care in the Community*. **10**(3): 196–205.

8   Gossop M, Marsden J, Stewart D *et al.* (2003) The National Treatment Outcome Research Study (NTORS): 4–5 year follow-up results. *Addiction.* **98**: 291–303.

9   Wright NM, Campbell TL and Tompkins CN (1999) Comparison of conventional and accelerated hepatitis B immunisation schedules for homeless drug users. *Communicable Disease and Public Health.* **5**(4): 324–6.

.

CHAPTER 11

The complex world of dual diagnosis, nursing and primary care

John Chilton

Introduction

This chapter considers the implications for primary care staff working with patients who appear to have both complex mental health needs in addition to abusing illicit and non-illicit substances. This is often referred to as dual diagnosis. However this term is now the subject of debate because of its impact on care provision and the fact that the majority of people may have more than two diagnoses that may include the need for social care, as the following quotation illustrates.[1]

> Substance misuse is usual rather than exceptional amongst people with severe mental health problems and the relationship between the two is complex. Individuals with these dual problems deserve high quality patient focused and integrated care.

For the purpose of this chapter, the term dual diagnosis will continue to be used to represent individuals with mental health and substance misuse problems in relation to the challenges they pose to service providers.

However, dual diagnosis *per se* does not formally exist as a definitive two-directional diagnosis and in 1996 Rostad and Checinski suggested that the term in itself could be interpreted as being misleading and cumbersome.[2] The range of needs presented by both substance misuse and mental health problems tends to be extremely varied and complex and if one of the problems were to be resolved, the other would still cause concern. In view of these factors, it invariably proves problematic to provide appropriate, well co-ordinated and integrated care for this client group. This results in individuals not receiving the care they should, in addition to them feeling dissatisfied, disconnected and disenfranchised with the care services at large.

Care services nationally have tended to adopt three types of service models:[1]

- serial
- parallel
- integrated.

The serial model implies that either the mental health problem or substance misuse problem would require treating primarily, before progressing to treatment of the other condition

The parallel model implies the simultaneous but separate treatment of both conditions. The patient would be required to attend a variety of services and engagement processes across the clinical landscape of mental health and substance misuse services.

The integrated model also involves the coexisting provision of both mental health and substance misuse clinical interventions, but supported by an identified lead clinician, specialising in dual diagnosis or a dedicated dual diagnosis team.

To date there is no firmly established standardised modality approach nationally, except for a number of 'good practice' template services, e.g. the compass programme developed in 1998. However, it is incumbent on local agencies to develop a service model that would deliver on the policy priorities set out in the *Dual Diagnosis Good Practice Guide*, thus ensuring a 'mainstreaming' approach to service delivery.[1]

How prevalent is dual diagnosis?

The prevalence of dual diagnosis is not easy to detect or evaluate. Many care services struggle in maintaining precise details on clients with dual diagnosis. However, in 2002 in the UK, the Department of Health estimated that about one third of psychiatric clients with serious mental illness such as schizophrenia had a defined substance misuse problem.[1] Equally, in substance misuse services, it was also estimated that about a third of the clients had some identifiable mental health problem, such as depression or an anxiety disorder.

Studies over the past two decades have suggested that a high correlation exists between high levels of substance misuse and complex mental health needs, primarily within mental health service populations across the globe. For example, in 1992 Cuffel suggested that individuals with schizophrenia were nearly five times more likely to have substance misuse problems when compared to the general population.[3] Indeed, a number of studies have demonstrated close associations between, for example, schizophrenia and substance misuse in terms of types of substances used as shown in the following list:

- 12.3% – 50% alcohol use (including dependency)
- 12.5% – 35.8% cannabis misuse
- 11.3% – 31% misuse of stimulants
- 5.7% – 15.2% hallucinogens
- 2% – 9% opiates.

It would appear therefore in view of the prevalence of dual diagnosis, in addition to the difficult and complex nature of the needs of individuals, nurses within a primary healthcare setting would inevitably have some degree of contact with this client group.

Brief profile of the common mental health problems

Some people who misuse drugs may find that they experience symptoms such as suspiciousness, agitation, emotional liability, paranoid delusions, perceptual distortions and hallucinations. These symptoms are also found in paranoid schizo-phrenia and can be exacerbated by illicit drug use.

Visual and tactile hallucinations are the most common symptom in drug induced psychosis. However, auditory hallucinations and persecutory delusions tend to be more characteristic of a functional psychosis.

A key feature of amphetamine induced psychosis is the absence of confusion and disorientation. Stereotyped or repetitive behaviour and 'picking' of the skin is a common characteristic of stimulant related psychosis.

Depressive symptoms such as low mood, sleep disturbance, poor appetite and suicidal thoughts are common in:

- alcohol dependency
- opiate and benzodiazepine misusers
- stimulant withdrawal.

Suicide, homicide and self-harm are substantially higher amongst substance misusers than in the general population. Irritability, restlessness and aggressive behaviour may result from either intoxification or withdrawal from substances.

Anxiety, panic attacks and phobic symptoms may also be precipitated by the chronic use of:

- benzodiazepines
- stimulants
- hallucinogens
- cannabis
- alcohol.

Difficulties in accessing services for dual diagnosis

Despite being labelled as 'chaotic' or 'troublesome', clients with dual diagnosis can be among the most rewarding to work with because of the many challenges they pose to nurses working within a primary healthcare setting.

Compared to individuals with a mental disorder alone, individuals with dual diagnosis tend to be more susceptible and demonstrate poorer prognostic out-comes. This tends to be characterised and influenced by a plethora of common factors with associated difficulties as follows:

- poor engagement with services
- unpredictable and violent behaviour
- serious and untoward incidents
- relapse and detention under the Mental Health Act 1983 within in-patient mental health services
- criminal justice contact
- vagrancy, homelessness and unstable housing
- family problems
- poor integration of care services
- poor compliance with pharmacological treatment

- poor diet
- increased risk of exploitation
- increased risk of contacting hepatitis B, C and/or HIV
- less likely to cope with the community at large compared to the serious mentally ill population.

Harm reduction model

The *Dual Diagnosis Good Practice Guide* suggests the use of a harm reduction model within clinical practice.[1] The model recognises that completely eliminating substance abuse would be impracticable.

Schneier and Siris recognised that a significant number of clients with dual diagnosis do self-medicate due to a number of common factors including:[4]

- self-medication use of substances to ameliorate uncomfortable/painful emotions
- negative symptoms of psychosis, e.g. use of stimulants to alleviate low mood
- neuroleptic dysphoria
- distress caused by positive symptoms of psychosis
- extrapyramidal side-effects caused through prescribed pharmacotherapy
- sedative effects, e.g. use of stimulants to combat against high levels of prescribed neuroleptic medication.

Case study:

Tom is a 25-year-old man who was diagnosed with schizophrenia two years ago. Over the past six months he has been smoking illicit amphetamine sulphate. He has experienced particularly strong sedative effects from his prescribed antipsychotic pharmacotherapy from his consultant psychiatrist.

Tom feels that the illicit amphetamine sulphate is enabling him to function 'more normal', and I can 'stay awake more'. Tom has not discussed his illicit drug use with his consultant psychiatrist, 'as I do not think he will understand'.

The principle of harm reduction aims to shorten an individual's substance abuse; but where abstinence cannot be achieved, treatment aims to alter the consequences of the substance abuse by reducing substance related harm to the individual and to society. This reduction in 'harm' to the individual could be achieved through a 'shared care model' approach, which would complement service provision in the context of treatment and service levels.

A shared care model of treatment is therefore a useful description of this approach and includes social care and recognises the importance of other professionals in the larger shared care team (social worker, voluntary agency staff, probation officer, health visitor, practice nurse, etc.)

Case study:

In the Gloucestershire Partnership NHS Trust, the dual diagnosis project is developing a 'shared care' working model (integrated model) approach to support individuals who experience co-morbidity. Nominated link workers from mental health and substance misuse services work collaboratively across both service domains, attending respective clinical meetings and reviews. Two pilot out-patient clinics at identified CMHTs within Gloucestershire are supported by the nurse consultant in dual diagnosis providing clinical consultancy/advice and monitoring of clients with substance misuse and mental health problems. Direct support to clinical staff is also provided related to dual diagnosis issues. The nurse-led clinics were evaluated at the commencement of the pilots at the end of 2004.

The aims of the project are to:

- deliver an integrated nurse-led service designed specifically for individuals who have defined co-morbidity problems
- work collaboratively with the CMHTs, developing standardised working practices in order to achieve successful delivery for the users and carers of the service and access to 'fast track' care and progressive care pathways
- widen access, contact and choice between the two services within a defined model
- provide an evaluation of the pilot projects which would facilitate the use and evaluation of clinical practices and interventions.

The advantages of a 'shared care' approach

- It ensures that treatment is accessible and relevant to the dual diagnosis population.
- It recognises the complex nature of dual diagnosis which does require a multi-agency treatment approach.
- It reduces the risks experienced by disconnected services and the population.
- It emphasises the importance for specialist care/treatment for priority clients.

Problems with a shared care approach

There are many opportunities for nurses working within a primary care environment to deliver care to those individuals who are affected by substance misuse and mental health problems. These opportunities would involve focusing interventions at reducing harmful behaviours which affect the individual who is experiencing problems caused through their problematic substance misuse and mental health problem. Examples of basic harm reduction interventions include:

- advice regarding safer injecting and avoidance of bloodborne virus transmission
- advice on local needle exchange schemes available within a locality

- advice on safer sex
- advice on contraception
- testing for hepatitis B and C
- vaccination for hepatitis B where appropriate
- enquiry about past drug use
- enquiry into other drug related problems
- enquiry into mental health problems
- liaison with infectious diseases services where necessary
- liaison with specialist services where necessary/appropriate
- liaison with mental health service where necessary/appropriate
- liaison with voluntary agencies offering supplementary services where necessary/appropriate
- liaison with dual diagnosis service where necessary/appropriate.

An understanding of the harm reduction model in the context of intensity of need matched to specific service requirement is advantageous in relationship to primary care for the following two reasons.

- Clients with a dual diagnosis with specific needs could be treated within a primary healthcare setting, supported by specialist services.
- Clients with a dual diagnosis with more complex needs can be referred on through clearly defined service pathways.

The primary care team utilising a harm reduction approach can differentiate basic needs with complex needs which will enable the nurse and GP to make appropriate referrals to secondary/specialist services.

Minkoff model

In 2002 Minkoff developed a model to describe the context of dual diagnosis by exploring the severity of substance misuse and of mental health need; thus the nurse within primary care would be able to plot service provision against actual needs (*see* Figure 11.1). This model could also be used within the context of assessing individual need in addition to determination of resource allocation and management, e.g. whether a 'shared approach' to care of an individual with dual diagnosis is appropriate or not.

The Minkoff model could be used as a 'triage' tool for example, enabling the nurse to view the 'differential' of need of the client in terms of where the client 'fits' within a particular service domain depending upon which quadrant they fall into. For example:

- *Quad. 1* Primary health care
- *Quad. 2* Mental health services
- *Quad. 3* Substance misuse services
- *Quad. 4* Integrated specialist team, or jointly worked by mental health and substance misuse services (virtual teams).

The model could be adapted according to individual service pathways in place at any given time. However, the nurse would be able to plot need in relationship to

Severity of problematic substance misuse

HIGH	HIGH/HIGH
e.g. a dependant drinker who experiences increasing anxiety *Quadrant 3*	e.g. an individual with schizophrenia who misuses cannabis on a daily basis to compensate for social isolation *Quadrant 4*
e.g. a recreational misuser of 'dance drugs' who has begun to struggle with low mood after weekend use *Quadrant 1*	e.g. an individual with bi-polar disorder whose occasional binge drinking and experimental misuse of other substances destabilises their mental health *Quadrant 2*
LOW	HIGH

Severity of mental illness

Figure 11.1   The Minkoff model (2002).

service allocation. In addition the model could be adapted into a triage/assessment tool. However, within primary care, emergency situations do arise most commonly with substance misuse problems, e.g. physical withdrawals, seizures, hallucinosis, delirium, tremors, self-harm, agitation and confusional states. The triage process may only last a few minutes with an aim to clarify the degree of emergency. However, the Minkoff model is an example of a practical tool that could be utilised at a primary care level within a simple formulation of practice ensuring appropriate access of treatment for the client.

Screening process

The screening process within primary care should be a standard practice for the practitioner enabling early identification of need for the client. However, the practitioner should always have an 'index of suspicion', especially for individuals with relapsing symptoms of mental illness in conjunction with substance use during the screening process. Mueser *et al.* highlighted a number of 'identifiable characteristics' which tend to be associated with harmful substance misuse and mental health problems that could be applied within a primary healthcare setting as follows:[6]

- young male – under 25 years of age
- episodic in-patient care
- frequent and varied mood swings on a line of continuum in the absence of a bi-polar disorder
- low motivation and volition
- exhibiting isolative behaviours in relationship to family, friends and peer group
- exhibiting suspicious (paranoid) behaviours
- exhibiting 'strange' thought or 'speech' processes

- exhibiting 'low mood' for intervals of time due to a lack of predetermined stressors affecting the individual within their environment.

However, the 'index of suspicion' can only act as a 'guide', and should not be adopted as a replacement for screening the client and as a 'stand alone' evaluation of perceived need/s. Rassool and Gafoor have suggested that screening a client should be facilitated within a safe, non-threatening, empathic, non-judgemental environment, ensuring that respect and dignity are maintained at all times during the screening process.[7]

Engagement

The development of a strong and trusting therapeutic relationship between the nurse and the client is significant in terms of engagement and the consideration and implementation of therapeutic interventions. The therapeutic relationship within primary care should be facilitated at a fundamental level. It may involve dealing with a number of intrinsic needs, e.g. confirming that the client is obtaining their correct benefits and that provision is made for them. Indeed, Gamble and Brennan support this approach and state that the 'strength of the therapeutic alliance would depend, in part, on the value a client attributes to the service. This can be enhanced by the style of practitioner/client interactions and by endeavouring to meet the client's initial needs'.[8]

In addition to the central importance of the therapeutic alliance, according to Capalan's theory of 'crisis intervention', is that as individuals experience crisis points, it can provide an opportunity for the nurse to support an individual to develop new strategies to address particular issues. He stated that 'crisis contains a growth – promoting possibility, it can be a catalyst, raising the level of mental health by changing old habits of problem solving and evolving new ways of coping'.[9] (p. 72) For example, a client whose symptoms deteriorate through taking illicit stimulants results in them feeling agitated, anxious and low in mood. Therefore, the opportunity for the nurse in primary care would be orientated towards presenting alternative methods of functional behavioural strategies and healthy educational advice in relationship to prevention of relapse in the future.

This focus on initial engagement with this client group is significant and of value within a primary care environment, which Osher and Kofoed have described as developing into a number of further stages that could provide a platform for interventions to be initiated either at primary or secondary levels of care.[10]

Stages of developed care

- Engagement
- Persuasion
- Active treatment
- Relapse prevention.

However, these stages do not necessarily develop incrementally, and invariably with clients experiencing dual diagnosis this tends to be a lengthy care process which will depend on the nurse's knowledge and clinical skills in relation to the area of dual diagnosis. The reality, within a primary care setting is that the initial engagement stage would prove to be the most effective stage. The practitioner's knowledge and clinical skills in relation to dual diagnosis would also impact on the particular stages of care which would be the basis for effective interventions with the client.

Screening/assessment tools

There are a number of reliable and validated clinical scales and questionnaires which could be used within clinical practice and the primary care environment by the nurse with dual diagnosis clients. The screening tools would elicit information that could be used as part of a risk assessment in addition to enabling the nurse to facilitate appropriate referrals to specialist services.

The screening tools used within a primary care setting should be short, concise and easy to understand for both the nurse and the client.

Examples of mental health and substance use screening tools

- **Drug abuse screening test (DAST)**: A 20-item screening test. The questions refer to a 12-month period of drug use.
- **Fast alcohol screening test (FAST)**: A short screening test which can be scored simply to determine risk.
- **Beck depression inventory (BDI)**: A self-report scale of 21 items which is used to measure symptom severity of depressed mood.
- **Beck anxiety inventory (BAI)**: A 21-item, self-report instrument designed to measure the severity of anxiety symptoms. The BAI overlaps minimally with the BDI.
- **Hospital anxiety and depression scale (HADS)**: Provides scores for depression and anxiety.

The scales could be used with a patient with co-morbidity, in conjunction with the screening and assessment of that individual. The information ascertained from these scales should not be used in isolation within primary care, but integrated and co-ordinated within an overall assessment by secondary care/specialist care services.

Urine screening

Urine drug screening is a comprehensively used intervention when testing for illicit substance misuse. There are commonly two tests, listed below, that tend to be used within clinical practice by the nurse to investigate substance use.

- Full chromatography test – urine sample is forwarded to a pathology laboratory for an accurate breakdown of metabolites within the urine specimen. The specimen tends to take up to four to seven days to process.
- *In vitro* test – saliva testing provides a practical analytical test result and can be used in 'user friendly kits' for almost immediate results, i.e. results may appear as early as five minutes. More information about saliva testing can be found on the

Altrix website www.altrix.com. Altrix is now a rapidly expanding company reflecting the growth in demand by criminal justice agencies in particular for this form of testing.

Detection parameters of common substances in urine screening

The detection parameters of substances are shown in Table 11.1.

Table 11.1   Detection parameters in urine screening

Substance	Elimination period
Alcohol	12–24 hours
Amphetamine	2–4 days
Barbiturates	4–21 days
Benzodiazepines	30 days
Cocaine	up to 3 days
Codeine	2–4 days
Cannabis	2–30 days
Methadone	up to 3 days
Heroin	2–4 days
LSD	2–4 days

Alcohol screening

A common test for alcohol abuse is the liver function test (LFT). This test will indicate whether or not the liver has been damaged through alcohol abuse. An LFT will detect enzymes released from damaged liver cells and the products of the liver. If there is a history of excessive alcohol consumption based on the screening process, an LFT should be provided within primary care.

A useful estimate for the nurse in primary care to ascertain current units of alcohol consumed by the individual would be to apply a simple unit calculation.

Unit calculation for alcohol consumed

$$\frac{\text{Volume (number of ml) of alcohol} \times \text{percentage of alcohol by volume (ABV)}}{1000}$$

$$= \frac{\text{number ml} \times \text{ABV}}{1000}$$

The result of this calculation could be used by the nurse to compare with Health Education Authority (HEA) recommendations for sensible consumption of alcohol for individuals within the UK.

HEA recommendations for sensible alcohol consumption for males and females
Male

Between three to four units of alcohol per day or less comprises no significant risk to health. However, continued consumption of alcohol of four or more units per

24 hours with no rest day within a given seven days would constitute an increasing health risk.

Female
Between two to three units of alcohol per day or less comprises no significant risk to health. However, continued consumption of alcohol of three units per 24 hours with no rest day within a given seven days would constitute an increasing health risk.

Withdrawal factors

The nurse within primary care should be aware of possible physical withdrawal factors which could also affect the mental health of the individual. Evans and Sullivan have highlighted a number of common factors that would require urgent nursing intervention.[11]

- Recent drug intake at levels that risk development of toxicity, poisoning or organ damage even if the individual appears asymptomatic.
- Ingestion of unknown quantities of substances.
- Opiate overdose – confusion, delirium, drowsy, unconscious, shallow breathing, pinpoint pupils, cold and clammy, blue hue to the skin.
- Tachycardia (if heart rate over 110 bpm).
- History of evidence of physical trauma (particularly head trauma).
- Individual is semi-conscious, can be roused but falls asleep when stimulus is removed.
- Severe withdrawal from alcohol and benzodiazepines – profuse sweating, shaking and tremor, high temperature and blood pressure, confusion, vomiting and nausea.
- History of difficult opiate withdrawal – runny nose and eyes, dilated pupils, goose pumps, shivering, diarrhoea, stomach cramps, muscle aches, clammy skin.
- Severe tremors.
- Hallucinations or marked paranoia.
- Blood poisoning – high fever, drowsy, red rash over the skin.
- Severe agitation.
- Poly-substance dependence.
- Seizure, or history of seizures.

However, not every client experiences withdrawal symptoms. Any intervention associated with the management of withdrawal needs should be carefully monitored by the nurse which should take place with the multi-disciplinary team in collaboration with the GP. Immediate advice regarding short-term management and treatment of particular withdrawal symptoms, if required, should be obtained by liaising with the appropriate specialist services (e.g. substance misuse/dual diagnosis services).

Screening of risk by the nurse

The screening and management of clinical risks in mental health practice has become increasingly high on the healthcare agenda. This has tended to be exacerbated by concern in society since the introduction of community care.

The resulting concern has led to the development of comprehensive risk assessment and management tools, such as the risk assessment management and audit system (RAMAS)[12], and of the care programme approach aimed at protecting individuals and the community at large.[13]

Indeed, risks do not necessarily present themselves only in the community. However, risk and risk taking tend to be common aspects of nursing professionals involved with clients who have mental health and substance misuse problems.

O'Rourke has described 'risk assessment' as 'a systematic collection of information which would determine the degree to which an identified risk would present or would be likely to present problems in the future'. The risk assessment and management of an individual should be aimed towards harm reduction as totally removing all risk within an individual's environment would be unrealistic.

Having a mental health problem would not be sufficient grounds for placing an individual in a psychiatric hospital against their will. However, there would be a number of conditions, beyond mental illness, that would have to be met before consideration would be taken regarding formal admission to a psychiatric hospital. For example, an individual would be judged to be:

- dangerous to themself
- incapable of providing for their basic physical needs
- unable to make responsible decisions about hospitalisation
- in need of treatment or care in a hospital.

The determination that an individual is potentially at risk is a difficult one to make. However, the nurse would have a clear responsibility in attempting to protect the community from potential violence to the patient themself and others.

The difficulty for the nurse in primary care would be to determine, in advance, whether an individual would be going to commit harm to self and others. Nurses tend to be on the conservative side when assessing for risk and consequently, an over-prediction of risk may occur. Practitioners tend to over-predict risk placing themselves in a 'no lose' situation. Indeed, screening for a general state of risk would not be the same thing as predicting whether a risk would occur. Risk would be difficult to predict because it would be determined as much by situational circumstances as it would be by an individual's thoughts and actions. If an individual disclosed thoughts or actions associated with 'risk behaviours' then the nurse should follow a number of guidelines.

- Is there a specific plan in place to commit self-harm to self or others?
- Are the thought processes related to risk occurring on a regular basis?
- Recent and past history of self-harm and harm to others?
- Does the individual have the ability to exercise risk behaviour?
- Has the individual been able to manage risk behaviours and cognitions in the past, enabling harm reduction strategies to be used?
- What are the prohibitive factors which have influenced the individual from not acting out risk behaviours?

The pressures on the primary care team would tend to be significant in terms of particular risk factors or associated factors, asserted by individuals with co-morbid problems. The nurse in the primary healthcare team should ensure that there are clear protocols and guidelines pertaining to risk that the PHCT and the multi-disciplinary team would adhere to in terms of 'standard practice'. The protocols would encompass all conceivable eventualities in terms of 'risk' within primary care, in addition to being evaluated on a regular basis, by the PHCT, ensuring that Department of Health guidelines pertaining to the care programme approach for individuals with mental illness are adhered to.[13] This approach would enhance the clinical governance of the clinical area, developing quality control measures and audit criteria within primary care.

The main aim for the nurse, when screening for risk within primary care would be to assess 'risky situations' as and when they occur, with the nurse intervening at the appropriate level as and when necessary. These normally include risk of self-harm to the patient, wider community or practitioner and provide a basis for breaching a confidentiality agreement with other agencies if more information is required to inform the assessment. However, it must be stressed that the nurse should never act as a 'lone' practitioner in terms of risk assessment, but should act with the multi-disciplinary team within the primary healthcare environment.

The development of a 'link nurse'

A 'link nurse' with special interest in dual diagnosis would enable the PHCT to provide a clear conduit between primary and secondary care. However, this would require further training (post-registered) for the individual nurse with special interest. The development of such knowledge and competencies within the PHCT would offer effective interventions for this client group.

Nurses within primary care could take a lead in developing the necessary skills and competencies within their practice. Additionally, actively participating in local project groups and stakeholder groups developing the dual diagnosis agenda within their care environment would be important in terms of bridging actual and potential 'gaps' between primary and secondary care services, aiming to deliver collaborative, integrated and evidence based service developments with individuals with co-morbidity and their carers.

Summary

The term dual diagnosis, or co-morbidity, does not have to represent complex and difficult care management by the nurse within a PHCT. Nurses increasingly will find themselves providing care for people with co-morbidity and complex needs. The phenomenon of co-morbidity is complex and does not offer short-term solutions. The consequences of co-morbidity, in terms of mental health, substance use, legal, social, physical and economic factors not only affects the individual but would tend to render society vulnerable.

Effective integration and communication at both micro and macro levels within healthcare communities (primary, secondary and non-statutory) will be key elements in developing dual diagnosis structures and processes that meet legal, professional and DoH standards, in addition to those of the clients and their carers.

The nursing profession is one major element in the response to the numerous challenges posed by this client group. However, nurses represent the single, and most prevalent, healthcare group providing care for this group of clients within the UK, which presents enormous opportunities and challenges for nurses within primary care, in addition to providing opportunities to develop 'models of care' that would be effective and evidence based.

At primary care level, nurses would be able to provide a number of clinical interventions that would be an important part of the overall clinical response framework. The screening and provision of brief interventions would be part of an overall harm reduction approach in addition to a brief assessment of risk undertaken by the PHCT.

References

1　Department of Health (2002) *Dual Diagnosis Good Practice Guide*. Mental health policy implementation guide. HMSO, London.

2　Rostad P and Checinski K (1996) *Dual Diagnosis: Facing the Challenge*. Wynne Howard Books.

3　Cuffel BJ and Chase P (1994) Remission and relapse of substance use disorders in schizophrenia – results from a one year prospective study. *Journal of Nervous and Mental Disease*. **182**: 342–5.

4　Schneier FR and Siris SG (1987) A review of psychoactive substance use and abuse in schizophrenia. Patterns of choice. *Journal of Nervous and Mental Disease*. **175**: 641–52.

5　Minkoff K (2002) CCISC model – comprehensive, continuous, integrated system of care model. www.kenminkoff.com.ccisc.html

6　Mueser K, Drake R and Noordsy D (1998) Integrated mental health and substance abuse treatment for severe psychiatric disorders. *Journal of Practice Psychiatry and Behavioural Health*. **4**: 129–39.

7　Rassool GH and Gafoor M (1997) *Addiction Nursing: perspectives on professional and clinical practice*. Stanley Thornes, Cheltenham.

8　Gamble C and Brennan G (2000) *Working with Serious Mental Illness: a manual for clinical practice*. Bailliére Tindall, London.

9　Coulshed V (1991) *Social Work Practice: an introduction* (2e). Macmillan Press, London.

10　Osher FC and Kofoed LL (1989) Treatment of patients with psychiatric and psychoactive substance abuse disorders. *Hospital and Community Psychiatry*. **40**: 1025–31.

11　Evans K and Sullivan JM (2001) *Dual Diagnosis: counselling the mentally ill substance abuser* (2e). Guilford Press, New York.

12　O'Rourke MM, Hammond SM and Davies EJ (1997) Risk assessment and risk management: the way forward. *Psychiatric Care*. **4**(3): 104–6.

13　Department of Health (1990) The care programme approach for people with a mental illness referred to the specialist psychiatric service. *HC(90)23/ LASSL(90)11*. Department of Health, London.

CHAPTER 12

Future directions and partnerships: the way forward for nursing

Rosie Winyard and *John Chilton*

The theme of partnership has reverberated through the chapters of this book. These include partnerships between the NHS and the Home Office at the most strategic level, moving to partnerships between drug misusers and primary healthcare team professionals at a local level. In this final chapter it is not possible to conclude these discussions about substance misuse treatments without coming back to 'joined up working'. However the balance of these partnerships may not always be equal. Influencing decisions for both service developments and developing treatments may not always be in favour of providers or service users, but may reflect a broader political or economic agenda on the grand scale of government policy making, both nationally and internationally.

There have been huge changes in some parts of the country in opportunities that have developed for patients to receive more treatments for substance misuse problems in primary care. This is partly due to the funding streams for developing treatment programmes that have been directed by government through local Drug Action Teams. Coupled with this has been a plethora of guidance and training initiatives from the NTA to improve the quality of services offered to patients from treatment organisations. Credit is also due to those primary care practitioners willing to develop more knowledge and skill in order for them to provide better care. Organisations such as the Royal College of General Practitioners and Royal College of Nursing run appropriate training courses, develop websites and harness enthusiasm at the annual national conference in substance misuse. It is now apparent that approximately 30% of GPs are willing to provide care for people with substance misuse problems.[1] But how far is this involvement going to continue in the future now that funding for forthcoming courses appears less secure, and to what extent can treatments in primary care be separated from involvement in the criminal justice agenda?

Does this change mean that more people are now able to influence decision making about drug treatments, including user groups, or is it simply the result of a government agenda encouraging treatment of criminal offenders with a view to reducing the number of people in prison for drug related offences? Only the future will tell us which one is correct and maybe both contain elements of truth.

The outcome of this strategy has come at an interesting time for primary care as it is affected by other changes in the way care is delivered nationally and locally through the new GP contract. In addition the shortage of doctors and nurses has led to new and innovative ways of working that have helped raise the profile of nurses and enhanced opportunities for the development of nurse practitioners, nurse consultants and nurse prescribing. Some possible future directions in primary care that may result from the advent of these new roles particularly in relation to increasing access to treatment services are discussed below, before coming to some conclusions about whether they are sustainable in the future.

Knowledge base of the addiction nurse

Every practitioner comes with a unique range of knowledge and skills drawn from their own life experience in addition to professional expertise. The following section outlines the key knowledge base that can inform the working of an addiction nurse in primary care (*see* Box 12.1). To expand this knowledge base requires a commitment to clinical supervision either individually or preferably in a multi-disciplinary group setting, particularly if the nurse is working autonomously and managed in a secondary care service elsewhere. Problems can emerge if there is conflict between the management of care between two or more services that may require resolution at a managerial policy making level in addition to good communication between clinicians.

Box 12.1   The key knowledge base in becoming an addiction nurse in primary care

Knowledge of:

- the local drug and alcohol scene with availability of support services for patients and their families, both statutory and voluntary
- what's on offer in the primary care setting – how to access help for drug related conditions and screening
- physical health, particularly pregnancy, sexual health and chronic physical conditions drawing on nursing and medical knowledge
- mental health, particularly depression, personality disorder and psychosis coupled with knowledge of the Mental Health Act
- public health, particularly prevention of communicable diseases, screening and reducing drug related deaths
- child protection procedures
- understanding the 'cycle of change' in addiction. Counselling skills and techniques including motivational or guided interviewing (MI) and cognitive behavioural therapy (CBT)
- evidence base of prescription treatments for drug related conditions, maintenance, detoxification, abstinence, relapse prevention and rehab. – advantages and disadvantages of these options
- local protocols for prescribing, supervision and recording treatments
- how to access local specialist services – referral pathways.

Skills of the addiction nurse

Competencies required by an addiction nurse employed in primary care are identified in DANOS competencies (*see* Appendix 4, page 181 for example job description). The role of the nurse practitioner in addictions can also be defined by these competencies in addition to those set out for the Highly Specialist Practitioner in *Agenda for Change*.[2] These criteria include a practitioner educated to Masters Degree level, specialist practitioner and management competencies relating to personnel and service developments.

Addiction nurses employed in current practice in primary care come with a range of skills (*see* Box 12.2) drawn from previous employment as general nurses, midwives, public health or psychiatric nurses. They are therefore highly trained, flexible practitioners drawing on a range of technical and therapeutic nursing skills with a commitment to working in the field of addictions. The skills they employ have developed by observation and example of specialist nurses or GPs, supplemented by training in addictions. In order to be effective in the future nurses need to retain an understanding of how addictions fits in to a changing primary care setting and continue to update skills in this front line area. This means working with whatever health or social care problem the patient may present in addition to their addiction as a function of the patient/practitioner relationship.

There may be resulting additional stress levels and 'burn out' experienced by addiction nurses and other primary care practitioners which makes it even more important to protect time for clinical supervision and reflection with other team members.

Box 12.2   Key skills of the addiction nurse

- negotiation
- listening
- communication
- ability to use and apply psychological counselling interventions
- developing a care plan in partnership with patient and others
- advocacy
- networking
- reflection, offering and receiving clinical supervision

- engagement
- observation
- offering respect and empathy
- ability to develop a care plan to include prescribing and flexibility
- managing resistance
- promoting self-efficacy in the patient
- recording information – IT

Training

Another important partnership is between academic institutions and clinical practice. There is a drive from the NTA to bring all practitioners up to an accredited level of skill in treating people with substance misuse problems. Nurse training provides a baseline of skill and knowledge that needs to be built on with a recognised course in addiction in order to develop a nurse professional body of knowledge in this area separate from, but closely allied to medicine and mental health. There are now recognised training courses, full-time, part-time and distance learning in addictions from Certificate to Doctorate Degree level at various colleges and universities in the UK, including RCGP training in the Certificate of Substance Misuse. The training courses include topics of prevention, treatment, criminal justice issues and management. All courses require the practitioner to spend some limited time in a placement setting, which may be primary care. In addition, substance misuse modules are often included in general nurse, psychiatric nurse, midwifery, medical or health visitor training. Debates focused on the limitations of nurse prescribing can often hijack a deeper discussion about other issues in relation to treatment. Many courses are now multi-disciplinary and facilitate a sharing of professional competence and understanding that can only enhance future ways of working in partnership. In addition, training and updating needs to be part of an on-going process of professional development in this rapidly changing field of health and social care.

The RCGP Certificate in Substance Misuse, parts 1 and 2 provide a good example of this approach to training combining two modules including theory with practical case management. This certificate is linked to continuing professional development and appraisal in order to provide on-going support and learning to GPs and others working in local shared care schemes.

The role of the nurse consultant and professional development

The introduction of the nurse consultant role has provided an unprecedented opportunity for the nursing profession and for individual nurses in the UK.

The nurse consultant role has four key functions:

- expert practitioner within chosen field of specialty
- professional leadership and consultancy
- research and evaluation
- education, training and development.

However, the primary focus of the nurse consultant is on clinical work, comprising at least 50% of the consultant's time; with 25% of the time spent on research in that clinical area and 25% educating others about the area of expertise.

Although nurse consultant posts are funded by the NHS trusts, approval for establishing them tends to be decided at regional level. The trust would have to justify the post within the context of the overall strategic aims of the healthcare organisations. The post ultimately will be based on clinical need and a 'business case' put forward justifying that creating the post would incrementally improve client care within the chosen specialist area.

The challenge for creating nurse consultant posts is to define a clinical area, e.g. primary care or dual diagnosis, where the evidence base for nurse consultancy is strong or the presence of a nurse consultant would measurably make a difference to clients' care needs. This is partly because of the time required to collect the evidence and also the difficulties in being able to identify and prove appropriate quality outcomes. Nurses aspiring to be nurse consultants would have to consider their career development carefully, because the created posts would not necessarily 'match' personal preferences or time spent in a clinical area without evidence of professional development.

The nursing profession generally has welcomed the opportunities that these posts contribute both to retain nurses within clinical practice and to enhance a career structure. This is especially at a period within the professions' history when at least a quarter of the most experienced nurses within the NHS will be reaching retirement age by 2009.

In the past, ambitious practitioners have had to move out of direct clinical practice, and pursue a management, research or educational route in order to develop their career and in doing so a significant minority has left the profession completely and pursued other careers outside the NHS. For the first time, however, in the nursing professions' long history, the maintenance and development of a clinical career structure would provide parity with other professions such as medicine and psychology.

Nurse managers, commissioners and professional leaders currently have a great interest in developing nurse consultant posts in line with the NHS plan.[3] However, they are also concerned that they may not be able to recruit suitable candidates. This is partly due to the lack of clarity surrounding the role and competing pressures in terms of commissioning arrangements, management disputes and continuing clinical demands. Unlike other professions such as medicine, which have a long and well established tradition of consultancy roles within healthcare, the nurse consultant role has a very short history – since the first appointment of a nurse consultant in 1997.

Developing expertise

There has been much debate regarding the particular characteristics of potential candidates for nurse consultant posts. These characteristics have been examined by Benner and Dutton who examined the 'novice – expert continuum' which could also equally apply to the development of any new nursing role including that of an autonomous nurse practitioner in substance misuse, mental health or nurse prescriber.[4,5] It is proposed that individuals develop through at least five stages of qualitatively varying perceptions of 'task' and 'methods' of decision making processes.

This five stage model emphasised the stages of 'expert' development along defined stages:

* novice
* advanced beginner
* competent practitioner
* proficient practitioner
* expert.

Dreyfuss and Dreyfuss pointed out that the different levels do not serve as a classification system or as a form of labelling, but could assist nursing practitioners in understanding their stages of professional development.[6]

As a perceived expert within their chosen specialty, the nurse practitioner is not expected to be perfect. They are able to demonstrate an 'intuitive grasp' of procedures based on deep tacit knowledge, not over-relying on procedures, protocols or guidelines within their practice. The expert nurse utilises analytical approaches when meeting challenges or can develop in innovative, safe contextual nursing practices. Significantly they are able to visualise what would be contextually possible within the care environment. The 'novice–expert' model attempts to distinguish the skilled behaviour of the nurse in relationship to the decision making that they process.

Nurse consultants as experts

In view of the descriptions by Benner and Dutton it would be assumed that only when a nurse performs at an expert level would they demonstrate the characteristics enabling them to function as a nurse consultant.[4,5]

However, there are numerous nurses who are performing as expert practitioners within healthcare modalities who may contemplate this career move, but be reluctant to take it because of fear of not being able to perform at an expert level. The 'novice–expert' model could be used by managers to decide on the suitability and appropriateness of potential candidates for the nurse consultant role. The model could also be useful as a means of selecting, offering support and training to nurses who may be interested in developing this career.

Over the coming decades within the nursing profession, theory, research and innovative practices will be produced by nurse experts. It is these experts that will create future developments, pose challenging questions for evaluating theoretical nursing and health paradigms generally. These nurses will play an important role in meeting the challenges, supporting and developing practice expertise, nursing research and policy making at a strategic local and national level.

The following section considers the impact of another key area of change on the delivery of substance misuse treatments, that of nurse prescribing.

Nurse prescribing

Traditionally the nursing profession has tended to assume extended roles, which have historically been undertaken by medical practitioners, e.g. blood pressure monitoring, carrying out patient assessment and diagnosis. However, in 1992, the then nurses' regulatory body, the UKCC emphasised the extended role expansion of the nursing profession, by increasing independent practices separate from medicine. Nurse prescribing, for example, is seen in the context of extended independent role expansion for nurses but is still subject to professional controls and regulation.

The Royal College of General Practitioners has endorsed nurse prescribing and has actively encouraged the development of prescribing legal frameworks to practice nurses, HVs or district nurses. This development has already had significant impact on the abilities of nurses' clinical decision making within primary healthcare. Extended nurse prescribing enables a practice nurse to use their clinical skills in relation to the patient's physical and mental health needs in primary care. This is in addition to managing any potential physical alcohol withdrawal issue and includes taking responsibility for the initial assessment, drawing up the treatment plan and prescription, thus providing immediate management and treatment of patient care. Currently some medicines to assist management of withdrawal from alcohol and opiates are included in the list of supplementary medicines available to be prescribed by nurses who have completed appropriate training. It is recommended that nurses only use their prescriptions in areas where they are already clinically competent and knowledgeable, although, like GPs they can potentially prescribe a complex range of medications in any situation.[7]

However until nurse prescribing is extended to include substitute medications of methadone and Subutex, the role of the addictions nurse remains restricted to often designing the treatment but being unable to fully complete the prescription, if substitute medication is required. Shepherd et al. suggest that nurse prescribing may not even be a 'genuine development' within a defined nursing role.[8] It could also be viewed as a covert attempt at decanting part of the medical role on to the nursing profession, thus limiting the nursing role in terms of patient contact which could impact on the therapeutic relationship with the patient. Other nurses would disagree, seeing their ability to prescribe as enabling them to offer a truly holistic service, completing a treatment package where prescribing is still only one aspect of a continuum of care.

The management and dispensing of prescriptions for substitute medication depends on locally agreed protocols that are based on the National Guidelines (1999). These usually include arrangements for safe dispensing with supervised consumption or daily pick up by a local pharmacist. Addiction nurses already have a key part to play in liaising with local pharmacists at the start of a prescription for substitute medication and its subsequent progress, monitoring effectiveness and any lapses. They may also be involved currently in issuing repeat medication or organising dispensing of this medication in blister packs for administration by hostel or night shelter staff. This is in addition to prescribing medicines for management of withdrawal including lofexidine and diazepam under a patient group direction. It remains to be seen whether independent prescribing for nurses will expand further to enable them to work even more holistically with patients who have drug and alcohol problems, and whether this does indeed increase patient satisfaction with quality of treatment and lead to improved outcomes.

Summary

The development of nursing expertise is therefore vital in terms of progressing the nursing profession, primary care and substance misuse treatment services. Crucially, the development of nurse practitioner or consultant posts will require significant support from Trust managers and others holding the purse strings for service delivery in order to develop sufficient numbers of nurses, with potential, to aspire to take up this role. It also requires these managers to offer continued support to practitioners when in post as they may become a target for unrealistic expectations from both patients and clinicians as they continue to develop their work.

Nurses are currently practising in a time of change, controversy and professional staff shortages. Within the coming decade, considerable changes in prescribing policy in the UK will occur as statutory and voluntary agencies, government departments and professional bodies work through many issues linked to nurse prescribing and the issue of patient group directions – *see* for example www.npc.co.uk/pdf/pgd.pdf. Currently diamorphine can be prescribed by specialist trained nurses in Accident and Emergency Departments and Coronary Care Units for the treatment of cardiac pain under a patient group direction, but as yet no substitute opiates can be prescribed for addiction treatments. The debate around substitute prescribing for opiates is one key aspect as many drug related deaths involve methadone. The fear of litigation around this issue has made many GPs reluctant to participate in prescribing for substance misuse patients. It is unlikely that nurses will willingly go down this path without generous pay enhancements that will enable them to purchase expanded professional indemnity.

In the future, if and when nurses can prescribe methadone and Subutex, many GP and nurse practitioners would still prefer to practise in partnership and consultation with each other as well as the patient, recognising the value of joint working and reflection that enhances treatment services.

Postscript

In March 2005 it was announced that a Bill will go before Parliament with reference to nurses being able to prescribe controlled drugs.

References

1 Substance Misuse Management in General Practice (2004) *SMMGP Network*. **8**.
2 Department of Health (2004) *Agenda for Change*. HMSO, London.
3 Department of Health (2000) *The NHS Plan: a plan for investment, a plan for reform*. HMSO, London.
4 Benner P (1984) *From Novice to Expert*. Addison-Wesley, London.
5 Dutton R (1995) *Clinical Reasoning in Physical Disabilities*. Williams and Watkins, Baltimore.
6 Dreyfuss HL and Dreyfuss SE (1980) *Mind Over the Machine: the power of human intuition and expertise in the era of the computer*. Free Press, New York.
7 Flint H and Scott L (2003) Patient group directions: training practitioners for competency. *Nursing Times*. **99**: 30–2.
8 Shepherd E, Rafferty AM and James V (1996) Prescribing the boundaries of nursing practice: professional regulation and nurse prescribing. *Nursing Times Research*. **1**(6): 465–78.

APPENDIX 1

Sample methadone prescribing protocol

Treatment for drug misuse conforms to guidance provided by *Models of Care*.[1] All patients referred to the addiction team receive a comprehensive assessment to develop an integrated care plan in partnership with the patient and other staff members. This enables a holistic assessment of their needs across health, housing and social care parameters. A treatment plan forms the foundation from which to set treatment goals and monitor outcomes.

The best evidence for substitution treatment in the drugs field is for oral methadone that has been shown to provide major harm minimisation outcomes in a variety of settings over a number of years, including primary care.[2]

- Higher doses are better than lower doses in retaining patients in treatment and optimising outcomes.
- Enforced reduction in oral methadone dose as opposed to maintenance is ineffective.
- Oral methadone accompanied by a non-prescribing intervention is more effective than methadone alone.
- The evidence demonstrates that methadone is effective in reducing mortality, reducing injecting behaviour, preventing people from being forced to commit crimes to obtain drugs.
- Treatment provided in primary care will be appropriate for many patients.
- Patients who may be unsuitable for treatment in primary care include those with complex mental health needs, young drug users under the age of 16 years, people neck or groin injecting, pregnant women. Treatment for these patients may need to be discussed with nursing or medical staff from the specialist services.

The rationale for prescribing either a maintenance or detoxification dose of methadone depends on the following procedures being followed.

- Patients must be registered with the practice on a permanent basis.
- Patients must be referred to the addiction nurse team for a full assessment. In exceptional, urgent situations it may be possible for a GP to prescribe methadone for a few days until the assessment date but this must be discussed with the addiction nurse on duty and agreed at the team meeting. In this situation the maximum dose possible is 30 ml methadone daily supervised consumption following a urine screening for assessment of illicit drug use, unless it is confirmed that a patient has already been receiving treatment from another GP or specialist provider.

The prescription of methadone is limited to 1 mg/ml mixture on a daily supervised basis. Prescriptions for injectable medication can only be obtained via a referral to the specialist services. Physeptone tablets may only be issued for patients travelling abroad who provide confirmation of travel arrangements.

- A full assessment should be completed including physical health, mental health and substance misuse. The patient does not need to come withdrawing from opiates as assessments usually take place in the afternoon. However on history taking, they need to report physical symptoms of opiate dependency and a physical examination should confirm the presence of needle stigmata. A consent form should also be completed in order to share information with other named workers in other agencies and a treatment plan agreed and signed up to between the addiction nurse and the patient. The information should be recorded in the proforma in the brown folder and notes made on EMIS.
- Prescribing should only be initiated after a urine test is positive to opiates and the patient is made aware of the dangers of using street opiates on top of the methadone prescription. The patient should be informed of risks of overdose and the effects of methadone in addition to the risks associated with interactions between benzodiazepines and alcohol. Caution should be exercised if a woman is pregnant (see the practice protocol for management of pregnancy). This should be supported by the provision of literature, e.g. *The Methadone Handbook*. Patients should be given the choice of methadone with or without sugar and the pharmacist contacted about taking on the patient for supervision before they leave the surgery. Patient identification or a physical description may be requested. The patient should be informed of the shared care protocol concerning information sharing between GP practice staff and pharmacists. Commencing titration, it is advisable to use a pharmacy that is open on a Sunday.
- Dispensing should always be on a daily supervised pick up basis unless the patient is working or for short periods around specific family or social circumstances and requesting a twice weekly pick up. In this instance it is only agreed providing the patient remains opiate free supported by urinalysis. These arrangements should be discussed for confirmation with the addiction team leader. When the patient is stable it is acceptable to collect Sunday's dose on Saturday. If a patient fails to collect their methadone without an explanation for more than three days, the pharmacy should contact the surgery and the remainder of the script should be cancelled. The patient needs to attend the surgery again for re-titration if they wish to continue with substitute medication.
- Recording prescriptions for methadone should be completed on EMIS by the addiction nurse or GP. Daily prescriptions are written on a green pad and need to be overwritten by the GP. Prescriptions should be written on a blue FP10MDA. The nurse stamps the script and writes daily doses in the boxes provided for a maximum of 14 days. The GP signing the prescription takes responsibility for the safe dispensing and administration of the drug. The addiction nurse takes responsibility for inputting into the discussion from her clinical observations and history taking from time spent with the patient.
- Signing prescriptions for methadone needs to be done by GPs who have been granted a handwriting exemption. If the patient is driving a car for work, the GP must inform the DVLA as described in the protocols folder.

- If a patient wishes to travel abroad and requests a change in their methadone prescription, 48 hours notice should be given. If they are moving to a different part of the UK, the same period of notice is required in order to attempt to ensure continuity of their treatment if possible.
- Titration should be commenced according to the level of street heroin or methadone the patient is using and is usually between 20–30 ml methadone. £5–10 street heroin is a baseline for 20 ml methadone. However, price changes and weight vary widely over time and in different regions in the UK in addition to individual rates of tolerance and metabolism of opiates.
- It can take up to 48 hours for methadone to be fully absorbed because of its longer half-life. The patient should be invited to return the next day or within two to three days maximum to review progress and increase the amount of methadone if they are still experiencing withdrawal symptoms that lead them to use street heroin on top of their prescription. Amounts should only be increased by a maximum of 10 ml at a time.
- Stabilisation with methadone can take up to two weeks depending on the patient's motivation to stop using other drugs on top of their prescription, mental health and housing situation. Once the patient is stable, other mental health or emotional issues may arise and need appropriate treatment.
- Methadone reduction is usually achieved by reducing 5–10 ml in a week depending on the patient's motivation to change. A rapid reduction can be achieved by reducing methadone by 10 ml a day if necessary, although this may result in extreme distress and should only be considered in exceptional circumstances, e.g. a patient requests it because of an impending custodial sentence.
- Local prison is now continuing methadone prescriptions for prisoners serving short sentences, less than 28 days. Other prisons usually offer rapid detoxes from methadone with Subutex or diazepam.

Prescribing is according to the NTA guidelines (2003).[4]

- Comprehensive assessment, review and multi-disciplinary discussion are required to establish a holistic treatment plan, set treatment goals and monitor outcomes.
- Adequate doses of substitute medication: 60–120 mg of oral methadone daily, particularly over 80 mg have been consistently found to be more effective than lower doses. Following assessment, this may require increasing to doses of between 60–120 mg of oral methadone for a significant time period (normally six months).
- Conventional substitution maintenance with methadone should be considered prior to considering an injectable prescription via a referral to the Specialist Addictions Service.
- A patient receiving a low dose of methadone, i.e. <40 mg, who refuses to increase their dose (e.g. due to side-effects) can generally safely transfer to Subutex whereupon higher doses can be used. Patients on higher doses (>40 mg) methadone cannot easily attempt an episode of Subutex treatment.
- Prescribing should be complemented by:
  - harm reduction services, including hepatitis and HIV screening and immunisation
  - support around social functioning, including referral for antenatal and mental health services

- structured counselling or other psychosocial interventions
- an expectation that the patient attends regularly for nursing and medical reviews.

References

1 Department of Health (2002) *Models of Care*. Department of Health, London.
2 National Treatment Agency (2003) *Injectable Heroin and Injectable Methadone: potential roles in drug treatment*. National Treatment Agency, London.
3 *The Methadone Handbook* (7e) (2003). Exchange Supplies, Dorset.
4 National Treatment Agency (2003) *Prescribing Services for Drug Misuse*. National Treatment Agency, London.

Sample Subutex prescribing protocol

Exclusion criteria
- hypersensitivity to Subutex
- acute alcoholism
- current dependence on benzodiazepines
- severe hepatic or renal insufficiency
- patients prescribed more than 30 ml of methadone.

Be aware
- presence can be detected by routine urine screening
- Altrix manufacture a mouth swab test[1]
- more difficult to supervise consumption.

Drug interactions
- CNS depressants including benzodiazepines, barbiturates and anxiolytics, neuroleptics, clonidine and related substances
- other opiate derivatives, including analgesics and cough preparations
- certain antidepressants, including MAOI inhibitors
- sedative H_1-receptor antagonists
- opioid analgesia is less effective.

Prior to prescribing
- referral to the addictions team for full assessment
- sample of urine to be tested for presence of opioids
- history taken to establish extent of dependence on opioids
- liver function tests may be necessary if history indicates abnormalities to establish baseline levels
- if using heroin, wait a minimum of eight hours before initiating Subutex prescribing
- methadone reduced to 30 mg per day, wait 24–36 hours after last dose.

Induction/titration

Rapid induction is the key to success. Methadone to be reduced to 30 ml a day. An initial dose of 4 mg will be required by most patients (the manufacturers, Schering Plough, recommend secondary dosing of 16 mg). They may experience some unsettled effects, particularly on day 2. This usually settles down on days 3 to 4 and they should be advised to continue their dose. If they use heroin on top of their Subutex prescription, patients may experience a severe headache lasting a few hours.

Side-effects for all opiates

- cardiovascular – hypotension, hypertension, tachycardia or bradycardia
- central nervous system – drowsiness, sedation, fainting, dizziness, vertigo, headache, euphoria, hallucinations, weakness, fatigue, nervousness, insomnia
- gastrointestinal – nausea, vomiting, constipation
- Respiratory – respiratory depression, cyanosis, dyspnoea
- Other – miosis, sweating, hepatic necrosis.

Most common side-effects include sweating, sleep disturbances and headache. It is more difficult to overdose on heroin due to the antagonist effect, but theoretically this is still possible. Patient information leaflets should be given with the initial prescription in addition to the Subutex medical card.

Sample induction dosing schedules

If increasing to 16 mg, Subutex needs to be introduced on day 2 or 3.

Day 1 (mg)	Day 2 (mg)	Day 3 (mg)	Day 4 (mg)	Maintenance dose (mg)
4	8	8	8	8
4	8	12	12	12
4	8	12	16	16
4	8	16	16	16

N.B. No patient should receive more than 32 mg of Subutex daily.

Maintenance

Subutex can be administered on a daily or alternate daily basis using a two or three day regime, although no more than 32 mg should be dispensed in any one day.

The effectiveness of alternate daily dosing is unclear and should only be considered in consultation with the team leader or GPSIs. Some individuals will not be able to tolerate two or three day dispensing regimes because they experience increased cravings or increased withdrawals on the days they are not using.[2]

Prescription writing

Prescriptions should be written on blue prescription pads with the supplied stamp, even if titrating the dose. More than one strength of tablet can be included on one prescription. Patients should be advised to attend the pharmacy for daily supervised consumption including weekends.

Pain relief

Paracetamol or NSAIDs, such as Nurofen, are first-line approaches. Avoid Nurofen Extra or any preparations with codeine. If further pain relief is required, this would need to be titrated in relation to the signs and symptoms experienced by the patient until an optimum comfortable level is reached.

Gradual dose reduction

Day	Dose (mg)	Day	Dose (mg)	Day	Dose (mg)	Day	Dose (mg)
1	8	11	4	21	1.6	31	0.8
2	8	12	4	22	1.6	32	0.8
3	8	13	2.8	23	1.6	33	0.4
4	8	14	2.8	24	1.6	34	0.4
5	6	15	2.8	25	1.2	35	0.4
6	6	16	2.8	26	1.2	36	0.4
7	6	17	2	27	1.2		
8	6	18	2	28	1.2		
9	4	19	2	29	0.8		
10	4	20	2	30	0.8		

Rapid dose reduction

Day	Dose (mg)	Day	Dose (mg)
1	8	7	2
2	6	8	2
3	6	9	0.8
4	4	10	0.8
5	4	11	0.4
6	4	12	0.4

Rapid dose reduction can be achieved over a 12-day period in which the daily dose of Subutex can be reduced by 50% every four days. This is suitable for non-compliant patients but caution must be taken that withdrawal symptoms can occur up to ten days after the last dose and may continue for two to four weeks.

Transfer on to naltrexone

Needs to be 48 hours after the last dose of Subutex and commence with 25 mg as a loading dose.

Transfer from Subutex to methadone

Methadone commenced after 24 hours after a 24 hour dose of Subutex and 48 hours after 48 hours of Subutex, then titrate methadone. There may still be some blockade effect on day 1 and patients must be advised not to take more methadone on day 1 in case this is happening.

Subutex dose	Initial methadone dose
Less than 8 mg	More than 20 mg
8–16 mg	20–30 mg
16 mg, or greater	30–40 mg

Overdose

Subutex is safer in overdose than methadone because of the 'ceiling dose' effect. It may occur in polydrug use. Very high doses of naloxone will be necessary – about 10–30 times that required for heroin due to the high affinity of Subutex for the opioid receptor.

References

1 Altrix Healthcare plc, Warrington WA3 7BP; www.altrix.com.
2 Royal College of General Practitioners (2003) *Guidance for the Use of Buprenorphine Treatment of Opioid Dependence in Primary Care*. SMMGP and RCGP, London. Revised in 2004.

Luther Street policy for the management of contacts with the addictions team

Patient expectations

1   You will receive treatment and counselling by appropriately qualified staff for drug addiction and also primary healthcare needs. Treatments may include substitute prescribing (with the support of GPs), psychological treatments, relapse prevention and motivational interviewing.

2   You can expect to be treated politely and courteously by other patients who attend for appointments.

3   Your addiction, physical and mental health needs will be identified in the course of an initial in-depth assessment where a treatment plan will be agreed and then implemented.

4   This plan is developed in partnership between you and your addiction nurse and will be reviewed at regular intervals.

5   You will be given a time you have selected from a range of options with the addiction nurse allocated to you as a keyworker, unless she/he is on annual leave.

6   It is possible to be referred on for further care and treatment, including mental health, detoxification at the Drug Recovery Project and other residential rehabilitation facilities.

7   Information shared in the course of your consultation will be treated as confidential within the Luther Street surgery, including the Drug Recovery Project if you are resident, unless it causes extreme risk to yourself or others including children. Information will only be shared with other agencies after obtaining written consent from you, if at all possible, unless it meets the above criteria.

8   Any information or data collection based on your contact with the surgery will be managed according to the terms and conditions laid down in the Data Protection Act and explained in the NDTMS leaflet available in reception.

9   If you are unhappy with the service you receive you can make any complaints either verbally or in writing to the Practice Manager or the Chief Executive, Oxford City PCT. In addition you can refer to independent advocacy services from Oxford User Team or the Patient Advocacy Liaison Service from Oxford City PCT. Leaflets are available in reception.

10 You will continue to receive appointments for prescriptions for methadone or substitute medication unless your behaviour is deemed to be violent or abusive, as set out in the Oxford City PCT policy on Zero Tolerance of violence towards staff. In these situations, appropriate procedures will be followed as laid out in the policy.

Staff expectations

1 The PCT has a policy of Zero Tolerance of violence and aggression towards staff and action will be taken to ensure staff, patient and visitor safety.
2 We do not tolerate using illicit substances in our practice. You will be asked to leave immediately, even if you have a booked appointment. If this happens again, a warning letter will be issued and further sanctions imposed.
3 We expect to be treated politely and courteously by patients who attend for appointments.
4 We expect patients to not be severely intoxicated with drugs or alcohol while they are present in the surgery. Booked appointments in the afternoon are for patients who are alcohol or drug free unless emergency slots.
5 Lost prescriptions will usually only be replaced on one occasion. The incident must be reported to the police before a subsequent prescription will be issued.
6 Urine tests will be required at regular intervals to support substitute prescribing treatments. For further information, refer to the Urine Testing Protocol.
7 Addiction nurses will always try to see a patient that presents on the day of appointment, even if not at the booked time. However, a prescription may not always be issued but you will be given information about how your prescribing treatment will be continued.

Appointment slots 'am' and 'pm'

• Eight morning appointment slots for all addiction nurses will be at booked times of 15 minutes from 9.30 followed by two slots available at the end of surgery for emergencies. Patients should make their next appointment before collecting their prescription and leaving the surgery.
• Afternoon appointments are usually reserved for assessments and will consequently be reserved in 30–60 minute sessions.
• If you are unable to come to your booked appointment and request an alternative, you will be offered the next available appointment with your keyworker. This may be on the following day. We will try and see you the next day if requested, but you may need to wait until the end of the morning or afternoon session.
• If you request an emergency appointment, this will be discussed with the addiction nurse on duty. You may be allocated a short appointment slot, if appropriate, or alternatively with a GP if the nurse is not available.

DANOS competencies for addiction nurses

Addiction nurse

Clinical standards – service delivery

AA Help individuals access substance misuse services
AA2 Establish, sustain and disengage from relationships with individuals
AA3 Enable individuals to find out about and use services and facilities
AA4 Promote people's equality, diversity and rights
AA5 Interact with individuals using telecommunications

AB Support individuals in difficult situations
AB1 Support individuals when they are distressed
AB2 Support individuals when they are substance users
AB3 Contribute to the prevention and management of abusive and aggressive behaviour
AB4 Contribute to the protection of individuals from abuse
AB5 Assess and act upon immediate risk of danger to substance users
AB6 Support individuals with difficult or potentially difficult relationships

AC Develop practice in the delivery of services
AC1 Develop your own knowledge and practice
AC2 Make use of supervision
AC3 Contribute to the development of the knowledge and practice of others
AC4 Support and challenge workers on specific aspects of their practice

AD Educate people about substance use, health and wellbeing
AD1 Raise awareness about substances, their use and effects
AD2 Facilitate learning through presentations and activities
AD3 Facilitate group learning
AD4 Develop and disseminate information and advice about substance use, health and social wellbeing

AE Test for substance use

AF Assess substance misusers' needs for care
AF3 Carry out a comprehensive substance misuse assessment

AG Plan and review integrated programmes of care for substance misusers
AG1 Plan and agree service responses which meet individuals' identified needs and circumstances
AG2 Contribute to the development provision and review of care programmes
AG3 Assist in the transfer of individuals between agencies and services

AH Deliver healthcare services
AH2.1 Prepare for the administration of drugs within agreed protocols
AH2.3 Monitor and respond to the effects of drugs administered
AH3 Supply and exchange injecting equipment for individuals
AH4.2 Support individuals in obtaining specimens and taking physical measurements
AH4.3 Support individuals and others to administer the individual's own medication
AH6 Prepare and undertake agreed clinical activities with individuals in acute care settings
AH7 Support individuals through detoxification programmes

A1 Deliver services to help individuals address their substance use
A11 Counsel individuals about their substance use using recognised theoretical models
A12 Help individuals address their substance use through an action plan
A13.3 Evaluate agreed group therapeutic activities

Addiction team manager/nurse practitioner
Clinical standards – service delivery

AA Help individuals access substance misuse services
AA2 Establish, sustain and disengage from relationships with individuals
AA3 Enable individuals to find out about and use services and facilities
AA4 Promote people's equality, diversity and rights
AA5 Interact with individuals using telecommunications

AB Support individuals in difficult situations
AB1 Support individuals when they are distressed
AB2 Support individuals when they are substance users
AB3 Contribute to the prevention and management of abusive and aggressive behaviour
AB4 Contribute to the protection of individuals from abuse
AB5 Assess and act upon immediate risk of danger to substance users
AB6 Support individuals with difficult or potentially difficult relationships

AC Develop practice in the delivery of services
AC1 Develop your own knowledge and practice
AC2 Make use of supervision
AC3 Contribute to the development of the knowledge and practice of others
AC4 Support and challenge workers on specific aspects of their practice

AD Educate people about substance use, health and wellbeing
AD1 Raise awareness about substances, their use and effects
AD2 Facilitate learning through presentations and activities
AD3 Facilitate group learning
AD4 Develop and disseminate information and advice about substance use, health
    and social wellbeing

AE Test for substance use

AF Assess substance misusers' needs for care
AF3 Carry out a comprehensive substance misuse assessment

AG Plan and review integrated programmes of care for substance misusers
AG1 Plan and agree service responses which meet individuals' identified needs and
    circumstances
AG2 Contribute to the development provision and review of care programmes
AG3 Assist in the transfer of individuals between agencies and services

AH Deliver healthcare services
AH2.1 Prepare for the administration of drugs within agreed protocols
AH2.3 Monitor and respond to the effects of drugs administered
AH3   Supply and exchange injecting equipment for individuals
AH4.2 Support individuals in obtaining specimens and taking physical measure-
      ments
AH4.3 Support individuals and others to administer the individual's own
      medication
AH6   Prepare and undertake agreed clinical activities with individuals in acute
      care settings
AH7   Support individuals through detoxification programmes

A1 Deliver services to help individuals address their substance use
A11   Counsel individuals about their substance use using recognised theoretical
      models
A12   Help individuals address their substance use through an action plan
A13.3 Evaluate agreed group therapeutic activities

Area B management of services

**BA Develop, implement and review the organisation's policies, strategies
    and plans**
BA1 Review and enhance your organisation's strategic position
BA2 Establish strategies to guide the work of your organisation
BA3 Contribute to the development of organisational policy and practice
BA4 Evaluate and improve organisational performance
BA5 Support effective governance

BB Promote the organisation and its services
BB1   Promote your organisation and its services to stakeholders
BB2.3 Respond to requests for information from the media

BC Deliver services to specifications
BC1 Develop, negotiate and agree proposals to offer services and products
BC2 Manage services to meet customer requirements
BC3 Manage change in organisational activities
BC4 Ensure your organisation delivers quality services

BD Provide a healthy, safe, secure and suitable environment for the delivery of services
BD2 Manage your organisation's facilities in relation to addictions
BD3 Ensure own actions reduce risks to health and safety

BE Manage information
BE1 Establish information management and communication systems in relation to addictions
BE1 Provide information to support decision making
BE3 Undertake research for the service and its clients
BE4 Supplying information for management control
BE5 Use information to take critical decisions
BE6 Prepare reports and returns

BF Manage the organisation's human resources
BF1 Develop a strategy and plan to provide all people resources for the organisation
BF3 Select personnel for activities
BF4 Develop teams and individuals to enhance performance
BF5 Lead the work of teams and individuals to achieve their objectives
BF6 Manage the performance of teams and individuals
BF7 Respond to poor performance in your team
BF8 Deal with poor performance in your team
BF9.1 Plan the redeployment of personnel

BG Manage the organisation's financial resources
BG1 Secure financial resources for your organisation's plans
BG3 Determine the effective use of resources
BG4 Manage the use of financial resources
BG5 Making and recording payments

BI Manage relationships
BI1 Develop productive working relationships
BI2 Develop and sustain arrangements for joint working between workers and agencies
BI3 Facilitate meetings

CA1 Identify the needs for substance misuse services and develop strategies and plans to meet the needs
CA1 Research the needs of the local population for substance misuse services in relation to homelessness
CA2.1 Support the development of strategies to meet local needs for substance misuse services in relation to homelessness

Index

Page numbers in *italics* refer to tables or figures.